Be Your Own Doctor
of
Health & Happiness

Also by Michael Lingard

Connection
"Towards a broader understanding of health in medicine"

Free Health
"Your own NHS – Natural Health Service"

The Buteyko Guide to Better Breathing & Better Health

The Buteyko Guide to Better Asthma Management

The Body Connection - eBook
The Guide to Better Body & Better Health

The Food Connection - eBook
Better Breathing Means Better Health

The Food Connection - eBook
"Let food be your medicine"

A Doctor's Guide to the Buteyko Method

Michael Lingard

Be Your Own Doctor of Health & Happiness

You *Are* a Miracle!

Lulu.com

First published in Great Britain by Lulu.com.

Copyright © 2024 Michael Lingard
All rights reserved.
ISBN 978-1-4710-9823-9

Contents

	Preface	8
	Foreword	9
Chapter 1	What Is Health?	13
Chapter 2	Two Views of Health	15
Chapter 3	Who are You Really?	17
Chapter 4	Are You a Machine?	20
Chapter 5	Are You a Miracle?	26
Chapter 6	Getting Started	29
Chapter 7	The Body Connection	31
Chapter 8	The Food Connection	37
Chapter 9	The Water Connection	44
Chapter 10	The Breath Connection	49
Chapter 11	The Mind Connection	56
Chapter 12	The Family & Community Connection	61
Chapter 13	The Environmental Connection	66
Chapter 14	The Earth Connection	68
Chapter 15	The Cosmic Connection	72
Chapter 16	Facts and Figures	78
Chapter 17	Swimming Against the Tide	81
	Afterword	83
	References	85
	Reading List	90
	Index	97

Preface

Why did I write this book now? There are times in history when, for reasons beyond our understanding, forces have gathered to allow major changes in society. I believe this is such a time when a critical number of people are seeking a radical shift in the way we live our lives. This could be wishful thinking on my part or just me dreaming, but a far greater man than me once said, "I have a dream" and it is no longer a dream, but for millions a new reality.

As you will learn reading this book, thoughts are the foundation of action and outcomes. We have to have a vision or a dream if we want to see change. Mankind right now has never been so urgently in need of a new direction.

This small book focuses on "health", but I have come to realise that health is far more than being well and fit, it is built on developing wholeness, *wholeness at every level from the sub-atomic to the cosmic*. The very origin of our word health came from "hale" the old English for whole!

My inspiration for this project is from two sources, firstly from all the work of past and present great writers I have been privileged to read. All I have done is made a small, rich cake from their ingredients that I hope you will find tasty, easy to digest and sustaining. Secondly, I owe my greatest gratitude to my late wife, Rosemary, for her support and encouragement for over half a century.

St. Bridget, Hawkhurst
July 2024

Foreword

Knowledge is proud that he has learned so much.
Wisdom is humble that he knows not more.
Cowper (1731-1800)

This above all, to thine own self be true,
And it must follow, as the night the day,
Thou canst not then be false to any man.
Shakespeare (1564-1616)

Seek inwardly the truths for which you yearn,
For you are part of Universal Mind,
From all the universe you shall not learn
Aught that within yourself is not enshrined.

Anon

I'm sure when doctors and health workers see the title of this book, they will be shocked, believing that I am recommending people go without ever visiting their doctor, or going without having any medical attention whatsoever! I would like to assure them and you, that this is the last thought in my mind. What I am proposing in this book is that we should all learn how to look after ourselves optimally, so that our need for medical attention is diminished greatly and that we can all live longer, healthier, more active, and happier lives.

This is not a pipe dream, way in the clouds woo-hoo, but is substantiated by the fact that all over the planet, there are "blue zones"[1] where the people there live long, healthy, active lives and hardly know what modern chronic diseases are. They have the secret of living the healthy fulfilled life that is within the grasp of all of us.

This book is based on over forty years of practising as a holistic therapist. In fact, it's my baby, which was conceived and has had a long gestation period of almost half a century. The idea that we could reverse the way healthcare is provided was triggered when, after spending over a decade as a graduate of economics working in industry and then as a restaurateur building a Michelin Star restaurant from scratch with my wife, I decided I wanted to train as a homeopathic doctor. After being rejected by a couple of medical schools perhaps because of my age, I sought the advice of our local homeopathic doctor. He advised me to get a medical training as an osteopath. I could teach myself homoeopathy, practising on cats and dogs! I was then advised by a London homeopathic doctor to train at the European School of Osteopathy in Maidstone.

A year later we had sold our restaurant, moved from Leicestershire to Kent and I had enrolled at the osteopathic college. I qualified in 1981 and joined forces with a number of like-minded CAM practitioners including an anthroposophical doctor, to establish the first holistic clinic in the south-east of England that year, The Wealden Clinic.

This multi-disciplined clinic was to be our training ground to help understand the power of our own healing abilities when helped with the appropriate therapies. Together we offered structural physical therapy, the Alexander Technique, nutrition therapy, acupuncture, psychotherapy, healing, homeopathy, herbal medicine, and more. At our regular monthly practitioner meetings, we would discuss, with the permission of the patients concerned, difficult cases which were not resolving well, and each of us would put forward our own suggested therapy into the pool for discussion. This was quite humbling for us all. I discovered that some patients with musculoskeletal problems, which I thought was my area of expertise with my training in osteopathy, could be helped better or faster with other therapies and, that this was the case with all the therapies. The challenge was finding the necessary support a patient needed to enhance their own healing abilities, putting our professional egos aside.

We should remind ourselves that man survived and prospered for hundreds of thousands of years with no medical attention, so there must be the mechanisms within all of us to deal with the hazards of illness, whether they be from viruses, bacteria, poisons, or injuries. The task we should be setting ourselves is learning how can we harness these innate healing powers which are at our disposal, rather than always trying to supplement or replace them with man-made potions and medical interventions. This would in no way negate the need for modern medicine and all its wonders but complement it. I personally would be the last person to suggest this, as when I was three years old my father died of a ruptured appendix at an early age because antibiotics were not readily available then. I am definitely not suggesting that we can manage with no modern medicine. It's all about finding the right balance.

Unfortunately, modern medicine originally driven by doctors dedicated to healing the sick and seeking better treatment for their patients, has now been taken over by the pharmaceutical industry, and the medical industry for profit and gain, as well as for the benefit of mankind, but at times the balance has got out of hand. We must now try to redress this imbalance, but that will not come from governments or industry leaders, least of all from the pharmaceutical industry, but must come from each one of us, with our own will to re-engage with our inherited healing abilities. In the next few chapters, I hope to guide you through a learning process that will lead you in months to come or even years, to become your own personal doctor! Let us remember what the origin of the word doctor is. I believe it was derived from the sense that it was a person who studied to gain more knowledge in any field, so we can have a Doctor of Philosophy, a Doctor of Engineering, a Doctor of Art, as well as a Doctor of Medicine. What I'm proposing is that you become a Doctor of Health and Happiness, not a MD but a DHH!

There has been a failure of modern healthcare and medicine to create healthy individuals, healthy societies, and a healthy planet. The remarkable advances in the treatment of diseases, of the technological wonders of diagnostic machines, and the rise of scientific research in every field of pathology that man suffers has not brought the rewards that should be expected. There is not a correlation between the increased resources spent on medicine and the resulting increased health of society.[2]

The leading country for investment in medical treatment is the USA with a spend of 17% of its GDP, but rather than being the healthiest society by all medical measures it ranks lower than other countries who spend only a fraction of that. The UK spends only 9% of its GDP and ranks 18th compared with the USA at 34th position. According to the 2019 Bloomberg Global Health Index ranking, Spain qualified as the healthiest country in the world with an overall score of 92.75 and only spending 11% of its GDP on healthcare compared with the United States with its overall score of 75 ranking 34th. Spain boasts a life expectancy of 83.5 years, which is expected to rise to 85.8 by 2040 and be the highest in the world. Spaniards eat a Mediterranean diet filled with healthy fats and legumes, fruits and vegetables, and less red meat and processed food. Spain has the highest percentage of walkers in Europe, with 37% of people walking to work instead of driving (only 6% of Americans walk to work). Additionally, Spain's universal healthcare programme is very successful and has lowered the country's rate of preventable deaths to 45.4 preventable deaths per 100,000 inhabitants.

This should surely tell us to look more closely as to how our government funds healthcare, health promotion and medical provision to benefit from a better balance between medical intervention, health education and support. As individuals we all need to learn how to take more responsibility for our own health by becoming Our Own Doctor of Health & Happiness.

Chapter 1

"There is a Ministry of Health, and a Department of Health. Surely, in the long view, this should be The Ministry, and Department of Public Happiness?"

Lord Horder (1871-1995)

What Is Health?

We are all reapers of a rich harvest of generations of minds far greater than our own when we express ideas, we often arrogantly think are primarily our own. It has taken me over forty years working in what is loosely called the healthcare profession, to begin to understand just a fragment of the real question that needs an answer, *"What is Health?"*

I suppose it seems so obvious to most of us that there is no need to ask the question? But when I posed this question thirty years ago to an audience of nurses and other healthcare workers, I discovered most of the audience couldn't answer it either! I asked; "Is it what was left after we have got rid of all diseases?" most of the audience shook their heads. Is the dictionary definition adequate? (Noun. According to the official definition of the World Health Organization, a state of complete physical, mental, and social wellbeing, not merely the absence of disease or infirmity.) They agreed that was getting better, but still not right!

Before the internet, as Socrates would have advised, when you have a difficult question we should go and discuss it with the experts in that field, but today we have Google, where I found an excellent comment on this question by Harald Brussow, [3] ".....Therefore I first went to health authorities like medical doctors and their authoritative textbooks that guided generations of medical students like Harrison's Principles of Internal Medicine. In the 18th edition you find ample material on pathogens, even a chapter on the human microbiome, a chapter on women's health, but no definition of health. Overall, one gets the impression that medicine deals with disease and not health. In a recent meeting, one of my colleagues said that the US National Institutes of Health (NIH) should correctly be called National Institutes of Diseases reflecting this disease focus of medical research. Health is currently fashionable as 'Global Health', but again scientists working at institutes like this, or in such programmes, deal mostly with diseases. After this disappointment, the author turned to PubMed, with 'health' and 'definition' as search terms and got less than 20 papers – a quite surprising outcome for such a central question of the human society. Clearly there is a problem with the definition of the term 'health'."

So, it seems I have not been alone in this quest for an acceptable answer to what at first seemed a very simple question! I believe one reason for this is that we all intuitively know what the answer is, but there is no way of expressing our inner understanding with just a few words. Hence it was my conviction that there was a need to attempt this problem by writing an entire book of over twenty thousand words to try to answer a simple three-word question! I hope, dear reader that you will find some satisfaction and resolution to this vital question in this small book.

Chapter 2

Two Views of Health

"One of the essential qualities of the clinician is interest in humanity, for the secret of the care of the patient, is in caring for the patient".

Dr. Francis W Peabody (1881-1927)

It is unfortunate that modern medicine has been primarily concerned with disease, illness and pathology for the past century and has not given the public much education and advice on health promotion. The main reason for this omission, is that doctors are not trained as health practitioners; they receive very little training in the fundamentals of health promotion: the need for good body mechanics, for good nutrition, for adequate exercise, good breathing, good relaxation, a healthier environment, and a supportive community. Because of this disease model of medical practice, the health system has become overloaded with an increasingly sick population, creating impossible demands on finance and resources. [7]

We have also taught an entire generation of the public to rely on their doctor to keep them well, and many people have lost their sense of self-responsibility for their own health or are just unwilling to do anything to help themselves. *Responsibility* is exactly the right word, as it literally means the ability to respond to any change and may have been the ultimate driving force of all evolution rather than Darwin's "survival of the fittest". [19] We all have this innate ability but may have been discouraged from using it when it comes to our own health care.

This personal *response - ability* has been usurped by the medical profession and by all therapists that have failed to help teach their patients to help themselves but have unwittingly made their patients increasingly reliant on their therapy for support. To be fair, to those doctors who have tried to motivate their patients, this may have been due their patients being unwilling to help themselves with lifestyle changes, as there is a prevalent view that "It's pointless worrying about our own health and quality of life or longevity, just carry on and enjoy yourself as we all die of something don't we?"

The truth is we can all have a profound effect on our health and longevity, and we can usually choose either a long, healthy, and active life or a chronically sick life for many years maintained with increasing medical and surgical interventions. The aim should be quality of life with longevity rather than longevity without quality of life!

If we in the UK follow the American lifestyle over the next few years we can expect the same outcomes. According to good medical authority we may be seeing parents routinely outliving their children for the first time in our history. It is now commonplace in America for young people to be suffering strokes or heart attacks and other chronic degenerative diseases that were usually found only amongst middle or old aged people in the past. The major reason for this catastrophic decline in health and increased premature death appears to be largely due to diet, lack of exercise, unhealthy lifestyle and increasing medical intervention with drugs and surgery. It is shocking to learn that the third highest mortality in the USA is due to medical healthcare! [8]

It was for this reason that ten years ago I decided to put all the findings after thirty years practicing in healthcare into one small book called "Connection"- Towards a better understanding of health in medicine. The conclusion that I came to was that our health depends on almost everything, even the cosmos! [9] This may have been the reason why doctors have preferred to follow the path they have taken, trying to fix or ameliorate diseases one at a time, rather than trying to teach their patients how to keep themselves healthy. However, there are just four factors we can all control ourselves, that can go a long way to promoting health and reducing the risk of developing chronic diseases or reversing them, which will be discussed at length later. They are our diet, our body mechanics, our quality of breathing and our mind health. *At the end of each of the following chapters you'll find an affirmation that you might like to consider using if it makes sense to you.*

Chapter 3

Who are You, really?

"Example is not the main thing in influencing others; It's the only thing!"

Albert Schweitzer (1875 – 1965)

This is a question that we don't often ask ourselves, perhaps because we think we know already, though that's not always true!

"Well, I am the physical product of my genes I inherited from my parents and ancestors!" *No, that's not true!* It would only be true if you had the same lifestyle, beliefs, and thoughts of your parents in the same physical environment! The new science of epigenetics has proved that every gene has to be turned on by our environment, our internal and external environment.[6, 52] So we can't blame our parents' genes for who we are anymore!

"Okay, so I am "my personality", how I relate to other people and events!" *No, that's not true either!* We are only consciously in charge of our thinking, behaviour, and actions for about five percent of our waking hours and ninety-five percent of the time our subconscious is in charge, and that was programmed mostly by our families before we were seven years old! Our subconscious brain can process over 20,000,000 environmental stimuli per second, but our conscious brain can only process about 40 environmental stimuli per second! [44]

"Ah! Yes, I know, I am the person in my body!" *No, that's not true either!* This will come as a shock to you and indeed to most people – your body is an amazing ecosystem that relies for its survival on a vast number of micro-organisms. Your own body is a community of 30-50 trillion cells containing 23,000 genes. That's not enough genes to produce the vast range of proteins and nutrients your body needs. It is estimated we need over 100,000 genes! Despite the fact we are top of the evolutionary tree we have fewer genes than many bugs or flies (a drosophila fly has 60,000!) Our genetic deficit has been made good by hosting a vast population of friendly bugs, bacteria, viruses, etc. that account for ten times more cells than we already have in our bodies, accounting for over 300 trillion cells if we are to be healthy! *So, in fact we are only partially our body!* [11]

So, who am I really? There is a meeting of ancient wisdom and modern science that is proposing the concept that our true self is our soul! This growing understanding has been supported with the advances in Quantum Physics and the "spooky" science that Einstein commented on. There is a growing belief that the fundamental "stuff" of our universe is not matter or energy but consciousness! You and your soul are part of this universal consciousness! You are not your physical body but far more than that, you are a part of universal consciousness that is timeless and spaceless. Now, that maybe too much to accept today, as it does take time for us to accept major shifts in our understanding – it took a few hundred years to accept the fact that the earth isn't flat! Perhaps we should all start thinking about trying to have a conversation with our real *selves*, chatting with our soul? [12]

Like it or not we humans are the product of millions of years of symbiosis with nature. That's how we invited all those microbes into our lives. When we live in contact and harmony with the natural environment we thrive. Our greatest error has been to progressively separate ourselves from nature in sterile, concrete, urban environments and even see nature as the enemy against whom we have to wage a constant war.

Despite the fact that of the known thirty million bacteria, only a hundred are potentially harmful, we attempt to eliminate all bacteria and other bugs with our antibiotics, industrial chemicals, the sterilisation of processed foods we eat and even with the cosmetics we use. If we are to thrive and enjoy better health, we all need to learn to live closer to nature in the future. [13]

The old saying that "no man is an island "is indeed true. We are all connected to the whole natural world and the universe!

That's who you are!

"I am the Universe!"

Chapter 4

Are You a Machine?

"It has become appallingly obvious that our technology has exceeded our humanity!"

Albert Einstein (1847 – 1931)

"Health is natural, disease is unnatural."

Anon.

"Osteopathy regards the human body as a perfect mechanism, all the parts of which must be harmonious relation to one another so united together as to form a perfect unit: otherwise, the body is in a diseased condition."

Dr. J. Martin Littlejohn (1865-1947)

Over a few millennia mankind has shifted from believing that we are but spiritual creatures temporally housed in flesh and bone, to our materialistic world view that we are biological machines that can be studied and fixed like any other machine.

It is true that there are many similarities between us and our machines, this is definitely the field of structural mechanics, yet another area that's been highly neglected in modern thinking in healthcare. Trained as an osteopath I have often been asked, does my back problem relate in any way to the stress and emotional problems I have been going through recently. I reply that I cannot separate the two, our mind governs our body and our body impacts on our mind, there is a total connection.

The grounding of osteopathic therapy and other physical therapies is encapsulated in the phrases "Structure governs Function" and "Function governs Structure". So, there is no doubt that we need to look at the mechanical integrity of our bodies in a way which we look at the mechanical workings of our cars and recognise any misalignments or malfunctioning structurally will impact on our whole functioning. We should attempt to correct these mechanical anomalies with whatever therapy we may choose. Perhaps I am biased, but the physical therapy that was founded to embrace the whole treatment of the patient was osteopathy in its early days. [10]

Just because there is a degree of similarity of our mechanics to that of a machine, we should not ignore the fact that there are far more dissimilarities. Our car cannot heal a fractured axle, it does not mind what we think about it, it can't deal with being "fed" the wrong fuel, it can't reproduce itself, it can't repair a scratched surface, and so on. But it is this materialistic view that has driven much of modern medicine. Perhaps the most serious impact has been the rise of specialisms with the consequent increasing attention to the individual parts whilst ignoring the whole person's functioning life. In earlier times the problems arising from piecemeal specialist attention was dealt with by the patient's GP who could help integrate the specialist's work into the overall treatment of their patient.

Today it is not unusual to find several specialists working on a patient, often unaware or even unconcerned of their individual impact on the work of their colleagues or on the overall health of the patient. In all professions there tends to arise a degree of narrow-mindedness or even arrogance that their own specialty "is the answer". This was the greatest lesson I and my fellow practitioners learned working as a group in The Wealden Clinic forty years ago. I like to think we all developed mutual respect for each other's specialty and learned the need to integrate all our efforts for the best outcome for the patient. The patient's GP now finds it almost impossible to understand the overall effect such specialist activity has on their patient or feels uneasy and ill-equipped to question the experts. Here is a major difference between the fixing of a machine and a person!

I am amazed at the foresight of the great physician, Lord Horder lecturing in the 1930's, and give below a few pertinent extracts from his book "Health and a Day" [14].

"Medicine has been mechanized like other spheres of action and the public has come to believe that machinery is revolutionizing the healing arts by dispensing the need for human judgment. It is true that the introduction of instruments of precision into medicine has been a great service, but the interpretation of the results obtained by them in the individual case still demands wisdom and experience of the part of the doctor. Where the machine is greater than the man the patient perishes. With the failing of reduction of medicine to machinery, the public seeks salvation in the specialist and the expert, and the more apparatus, and the more complicated employed by these specialists, the greater his confidence.

On waking in the night with a pain in the belly, the patient's immediate anxiety is not whether he will find his physician available, but whether the right specialist is sent for. Is it the appendix, or the gallbladder, or the stomach, or the kidney man he needs call? What if he rings up the wrong one? Perhaps the trouble isn't in his belly at all, for suddenly he remembers that what his business friend thought was a severe attack of indigestion last week turned out to be a coronary thrombosis. So perhaps it is the cardiologist he needs. God! How difficult life - and especially medicine - is!

With the growth of specialisms have appeared the diagnostic clinic and group medicine practices, undoubtedly the group system has its advantages. But there is the point at which, after a complete history of the case is obtained and a general and thorough overhaul is made, the decision is arrived at as to what special examination shall be undertaken. Then there is a point at which the correlation and interpretation of the results of such special examinations are considered in relation to the patient. If there is no assessor, that used to be the patient's GP whose duty it was to assess these two important functions, the whole system breaks down.

Regarding the first, a sensitive and apprehensive patient may easily be made still more so by elaborate investigations which are not really indicated, or an invalid may be produced who previously did not exist. Regarding the second point the danger is equally great. Patient dossiers are apt in these days to be so full and so heterogeneous that only the wisest clinician might be sensitive to what is most significant. The exercise of this sensitiveness becomes more and more essential the more meticulously exact reports of the experts may be. These reports tend to be more and more meticulously exact with the increasing tendency to specialism and the myopia that goes with it. The number of patients whose hearts are healthy is in inverse proportion to the number of cardiologists they consult, and the frequency of which they are "electrocardiographed". An upper respiratory tract which is passed as "normal" by careful 'nose and throat man' will soon be so rare as to merit demonstration at the Academy of medicine. Someone must preserve his poise and if the clinician does not, no one does.

The way of health is pictured as a tightrope along which we make a slow and intrepid progress. The least shift to left or right, not immediately corrected or corrected inaccurately, and we are plunged headlong into the abyss of disease. Here await his inflammations and ulcers and cancer, especially cancer. Of all the people who disseminate these ideas the worst enemies are those of the medical profession because they are thought to speak with authority. It is for the general clinician to prick this kind of bubble and to point out that health is really a broad and well paved road. And, speaking generally, and given a modicum of good fortune, the wayfaring man should enjoy good health. Again, if the physician drops out there is no one left to make real contact with the patient on the psychological side.

What all this boils down to is the plea for the maintenance of the family physician, the General practitioner, that is. This spread of specialisms and this interest of the public in medical matters have combined to narrow the function of the General practitioner, who is, or who should be, the clinician par excellence, almost to the vanishing point. I regard this as being no less dangerous to the public than it would be for the passengers of the ship, if the captain left the bridge and the chief engineer, or the chief steward or the radio operator, took his place. But I see the equivalent of this being done day after day. Whereas formerly the physician kept control of the case and exercised his judgment in deciding the programme of treatment, he now, all too often, stands aside and allows his specialist colleagues to take charge, over the shoulders of whom as it were, he gets an occasional and momentary glimpse of his patient. The specialist is there from the first one or a number, for it is not uncommon to see a patient being treated by a committee, just as though he were a banking concern, run by a board of directors; only the patient is in a worse plight, because even the bank has its manager.

Meanwhile the patient's own knowledge has expanded in the medical field so that he knows a lot of technical terms and quite often he can no longer tell the doctor of his symptoms in plain language. What's the matter with you we ask him. "Blood pressure, doctor" he replies. 'No, but what are you suffering from?' "I told you doctor, blood pressure". And since we must make a beginning somehow, we say 'Yes, but tell me how it is affecting you.' "Oh, you mean my giddiness', or 'my headache', and at last we are back at scratch.

He carries the electrocardiographic tracing about with him and points out to as the deviation of the T wave from the accepted normal. The X-ray pictures of his opaque meal have preceded his visit some of the results of the biochemical research duly recorded with zeal, more excessive than commendable on a form of enormous size. And if we gently push these things aside, and ask him a few simple questions, and then examine him with our unaided senses, he thinks our methods are medieval. He little knows how ultra-modern they really are... We never should have left the bedrock of clinical medicine. And the sooner we return to it the better." Lord Horder [14]

It may have been reading those words of Lord Horder above, that initially prompted me to set pen to paper for this book. I fear that his hope for a return to medical sanity may never be, that the General Practitioner of old will not be re-instated to his rightful position, and that the trend to more reductionism and the loss of personalised individual medicine will continue.

It is for this reason that I believe we must all begin to assume that demanding role of being Our Own Doctor of Health & Happiness! I am aware that this role should be restricted to whatever we can do ourselves to change our lifestyle, to enhance our health and wellbeing, as, like the GP of old, we shall not be able to assess the optimal medical specialist intervention.

All that we will be able to do will be to resist medical intervention whenever there is an alternative, that is scientifically proven or that we judge of sufficient anecdotal strength to help us, be it for minor maladies or serious chronic diseases. This is not new, there are many patients who are not satisfied with only "the current medical protocol and diagnosis" and are doing their own research and seeking support from others in their position who have demonstrated the value of natural remedies or lifestyle changes.

In time, I am hopeful that the medical profession will be supportive of this growing development of individual patient responsibility for their own health, if only because of the almost exponential growth of medical intervention costs for individuals and society. Only when the public are educated and supported by their own doctor or specialist to take more responsibility will this be possible.

Currently, those foreword looking GPs who have attempted the engagement of the patient in changing their lifestyle have too often met with rejection. "No, doctor! Can't you give me some medicine to fix this problem, I don't want to change my lifestyle?" This attitude of the patient must change if we are to gain the greatest benefit from both modern medicine and our individual lifestyle changes.

This is my argument for you and I being your Own Doctor of Health & Happiness.

"I am a miraculous machine!"

Chapter 5

You are a Miracle.

"There are only two ways to live your life. One way is as though nothing is a miracle. The other way is as though everything is a miracle".

Albert Einstein (1879-1955)

It sometimes pays to stop and think and take note of where we are and who we are to gain a sense of the miraculous. You and I have inherited the evolutionary miracle over thousands of years from single celled creatures through all ranges of invertebrates, mammals, and others to the point where today we see ourselves at the top of this evolutionary tree.

Over those thousands of years or even longer we have developed a means of living, a means of survival and the means of thinking that deserves a little more attention. Much of this incredible development has been due to a single concept that I like to consider, namely, *response-ability.* Yes, it has been throughout those vast periods of time, our *ability to respond to our environment* that has driven our ever-successful evolution. Remember that this process of evolution has not stopped and that we are still very much in this process each one of us in our own lives.

So, what has this evolution given us as human beings? Perhaps the essence of this small book is attempting to answer this major question. It would be difficult to argue that we have not developed a remarkable ability to ward off and conquer diseases wherever they come from, otherwise we would not be here to tell the story. It would be difficult to argue that we have not evolved to understand how to live in our environment and thrive, otherwise you would have not reached this stage of our development. It would be difficult to argue that we have not evolved an ability to think beyond the mere necessity of survival, otherwise we would not have developed all the mental skills and abilities in science and art that we enjoy today.

For most of this journey as humans we had no medical support in this process of survival, which surely means that we all have all the necessary abilities to live long and healthy lives so long as we learn to respond intelligently to our environment, so long as we become *response-able* individuals. This is no simple achievement as it will include evaluating all those things in our environment that maybe affecting us adversely or beneficially and choosing the right ones to correct, avoid or enhance.

I'm sure for primitive man this was almost second nature. Some have argued that this is exactly why we have developed our large, complex brain. As hunter-gatherer we had to have a truly encyclopaedic knowledge of our fauna and flora, which leaves, berries, shoots or roots were good to eat and which were poisonous, how to track down animals, grubs or insects that could be caught or found without too much effort, how to shelter from the seasonal changes of weather and how to avoid even invisible health hazards of diseases. Sadly, modern man has lost conscious awareness of this encyclopaedic knowledge and has increasingly become reliant on our survival with advice and direction of others, and especially to modern medical intervention with drugs or surgical work. We have almost entirely lost our ability to respond intelligently to our environment, we have become *irresponsible!*

The good news is that despite our loss of *response-ability* we still have all those ancient inherent abilities to use and support our daily lives. This is the miraculous legacy we all have, our innate healing powers to repair tissue damage, to combat harmful viruses or bacteria, to extract all the complex nutrients from our food and deliver exactly the nutritional requirements to every specialised cell in our bodies, to maintain our body temperature, our blood circulation, our breathing at just the right levels and far more. All this with the integration and help from the thousands of beneficial bacteria, viruses, and other micro-organisms that we all naturally host. We must all start to become more aware of our miraculous capacity for healthy living and to support it in our lifestyle. This does not mean we should reject all our modern discoveries in healthcare, but we can enjoy both our inherited capabilities and our modern aids. Surely this would be a win-win approach.

There is a growing body of well documented, scientifically tested "spontaneous remissions", patients recovering from "incurable diseases" without medical intervention. This perhaps demonstrates the extreme impact of this miraculous healing potential we all have. I am not suggesting this extreme example of self-help is within the ability or acceptability of everyone, but it should encourage us all to ponder just how much we could help ourselves to simply lead a healthier, happier, longer active lives if we only tweaked our lifestyles a little. [20] [21]

"I am a Miracle!"

Chapter 6

Getting Started

"Nothing will benefit human health and increase the chances for survival of life on earth as much as the evolution to a vegetarian diet."

Albert Einstein (1879 - 1955) [38]

Change is always a challenge that is usually accompanied with many questions both anxiety-provoking as well as uplifting and positive. When it comes to lifestyle changes each one of us will have initial reservations as to how far we are willing to change our daily life. It will in the end be a compromise we accept on a day by day, week by week process of trial and error. Some may begin just making minor changes others may decide it is worth taking a leap of faith and accepting major changes to quickly establish the potential benefits.

These changes discussed in the following chapters are based on a book I published some years ago entitled "Connection" - towards a broader standing of health in medicine. [5]

I set out to find the key factors that appear to be connected to promoting health and avoiding disease. As we have already seen, it is far easier to study those factors that contribute to disease, but harder to identify those that enhance our health, since we are only intuitively aware of what health is!

Each key factor is, and always will be, cause for discussion and a challenge to find any consensus, or evidence. Rather than spend time on this debate I have tried to follow what at this time appear to be well founded choices. Roughly speaking we deal with: The Body Connection, The Food Connection, The Breath Connection, The Mind Connection and other less obvious but vitally important connections.

It is unfortunate that modern medicine has been primarily concerned with disease, illness and pathology and has not given the public much advice on health promotion. The main reason for this omission, is that doctors are not trained as health practitioners, they receive very little training in the fundamentals of health promotion: the need for good body mechanics, for good nutrition, for adequate exercise, good breathing, good relaxation, a healthy environment, and a supportive community. When I was a member of The Royal Institute of Medicine, I visited their extensive library to see what books they had on the vital subject of "health". I was disappointed but not surprised that I found very few, and even those I found dealt with the subject of "disease prevention" with vaccination etc. which is a negative viewpoint. When I left, I donated two books to help redress this imbalance: "The China Study" by Dr. T. Colin Campbell, and my own small book "Connection"- Towards a broader understanding of health in medicine. Because of this predominant disease model of medical practice, our healthcare systems are overloaded with a sick population that is creating increasingly impossible demands on finance and resources.

We also have encouraged an entire generation to rely on their doctor to keep them well and who have lost their sense of self-responsibility for their own health, or they are just unwilling to do anything to help themselves. The truth is we can have a profound effect on our health and longevity, and we can usually choose for either *a long healthy active life with minimal medical interventions, or an equally long but chronically sick life with maximum medical interventions.*

The following chapters will offer you positive lifestyle changes that will improve your health and wellbeing and reduce the risks of developing chronic diseases or even reverse many established diseases. It will give you the chance to evaluate your current lifestyle and compare it with potential improvements you could make.

I hope you benefit greatly from this journey of discovery and wish you "Bon Voyage!"

"I am set and ready for the journey!"

Chapter 7

The Body Connection

"Structure governs Function, Function governs Structure."
"The rule of the artery reigns supreme."

Anon.

We are only recently discovering the almost infinite complexity of the human body; it is perhaps the most amazing "machine" in the universe and yet mainstream medicine has not recognised this when health is affected by structural problems. Every machine obeys the same laws of mechanics, a minor misalignment or restriction of a part of a watch or car will have serious effects on its functioning, with parts wearing out, abnormal working or complete cessation.

However, it appears, that in modern medicine, dominated by drug therapy and reductionism, there is a belief that the human body is "oddly unique", in that it will function well regardless of its structural alignment, with perhaps the exception of fractures or dislocations. Once we accept the above it follows that the reverse is true that any disturbed function or abnormal activity will have an adverse effect on the structure of the body from minor local irritation to major pathologies. The body structure is a unity and, it may not be an exaggeration to say, that every cell in our bodies is connected in some way to every other cell. It is easy to understand that, like the old song says, "the head bone is connected to the neck bone, the neck bone is connected to the shoulder bone..." every bone is connected to every other bone. Thus, any mechanical problem in one area of the body will produce an effect throughout the entire body. A painful foot will cause one to limp, the awkward abnormal gait will strain the whole back, causing internal organ dysfunction and even more.

The body heals itself if conditions are right. It has often been said the physician treats, but the body heals. The human body is always working to maintain a state of balanced function. Physical examinations and lab tests are designed to measure those physiologic activities the body keeps constant: blood pressure, blood sugar, heart rate, etc. that should all stay within a normal range. The body remains balanced in three-dimensional space. We can stand on one foot, hold a book in one hand, read, and at the same time bring a cup to our lips without even looking, and without falling over. This is a complex task requiring a constant self-correcting mechanism. When a patient suffers a laceration, a physician can only assist by cleaning the wound, and bringing the edges together. The healing occurs on its own. There is within each of us an inherent healing functionality that constantly works to restore homeostasis and body integrity. An integral part of this self-healing process is found in the arterial circulation of the blood. When blood and lymphatics flow freely, tissues can perform their physiologic functions normally. With the occurrence of any trauma, physical or emotional, the tissues contract, twists, and compresses and the fluid flow becomes obstructed. This can then become a significant contributor to the onset of disease. Mechanical adjustment restores freedom in the tissue, normalizes fluid flow and thus the inherent physiologic function of healing.

Every cell in our body requires nutrition, oxygen and protection from foreign viruses or bacteria. The arterial blood carries all these components to every cell where physically possible; it is the vital internal environment. Restriction of arterial blood flow either by physical compression of the blood vessels or by the contraction of smooth muscle tissue from nerve root irritation, is perhaps a prime factor in all diseases. *It was the recognition of this process that led to the development of osteopathy as a total medical system over a century ago and has since been the basis of all positive results of physical therapy.*

Over the years there has been a tendency for the public to regard osteopathy and other physical therapies akin to osteopathy to be primarily for bad backs, and not a valuable aid to support any other therapy for almost any other condition. In part, this has been due perhaps to the acceptance by some in the profession to restrict their activity specifically to the basic treatment of back problems with their patients, and in part due also to the lack of understanding on the part of the wider medical fraternity of the power of physical treatment aiding healing and recovery. The remit and scope of osteopathic treatment is dependent on the training and aims of the individual therapist. Some therapists have expanded their range of treatment modes to cranial osteopathy, functional release work, posture correction, and dare I even say it, psychological impact on the body.

I wonder how many people would consider any of the following situations for visiting an osteopathic practitioner: an irritable baby troubled with colic and poor sleep, a person with long-standing discomfort and restriction following a simple strained ankle, a young person with crooked or crowded teeth, a person opting for osteopathic help for a chronic knee problem rather than a replacement joint, a person with recurrent gut problems not responding to medicine or a migraine sufferer? All these conditions may be helped or resolved if closely related to structural problems.

What can you do yourself to improve your body mechanics? The truth is, once your mechanics have become seriously compromised with misalignments, restrictions, or complex accommodation to structural faults, you, like me, will need to get help from a physical therapist. Much as I would like it, *I can't adjust my own structure with my own structure!*

The following exercises can be useful to keep your mechanics in order:

Checking Your Pelvis is Level:

When the pelvis torsions it causes the hip joints to rotate in a way that you can see when lying on your back on the floor. Lay flat on the floor with your legs straight and notice whether your feet are placed symmetrically. If your right foot rolls out further than your left foot it usually indicates your pelvis is twisted - your pelvis has gone forward on your right and backwards on your left. This may be due to restrictions in your lumbar vertebrae that will need structural attention.

The Pisa Pelvic Exercise:
If your pelvis appears level or after you have had structural treatment to make it so, you can help keep it from tilting in the future with this simple thirty second daily exercise. This exercise involves lying on your back taking hold of your *right* knee and pulling with both hands towards your chest sufficient to stretch the posterior muscles and ligaments on your right side of your pelvis for just thirty seconds, then release. End of exercise!

I began by trying this on myself, and now can maintain a level pelvis this way for over a year, which is good for me as before I used to need a treatment and a pelvic adjustment every few months. There are no adverse side effects, except it might affect your osteopath's business adversely, as you will be able to go longer between treatments! Simple to do in bed or lying in your bath so why not try it yourself and even tell your friends about it, I do.

Remember this is *intentionally an asymmetric exercise* just on the *right, as almost 99% of pelvic twists are forward on the right, you will need to listen to my podcast:* "The Pisa Pelvic Exercise"[50] *to understand why!*

The Sub-occipital Release: (Two old tennis balls in a sock)
To help relaxation or to reduce a stress headache, this exercise reduces the tension at the base of the skull, thereby reducing irritation to the large vagus nerve and improving circulation of blood to the head. You will need two soft old tennis balls, pushed into a sock and the end of the sock tied to keep them together.

Lay flat on the floor with the tennis ball sock under your skull as a pillow, allow your head to relax like this for a few minutes then sit up. The gentle pressure on the pair of occipital bones at the base of your skull are compressed causing a shift of cerebral-spinal fluid throughout your nervous system whilst stretching all the tense muscles at the base of your skull. WARNING: Do not use this exercise if you have any cardio-vascular problem.

Stretching Exercises:

We naturally often find ourselves stretching without thinking, it is the body's way of reducing tension or improving muscle functioning. Thus, any stretching exercises you find suit you, or you can fit into your daily routines will be beneficial. The secret is to try to maintain fullest mobility by gently extending the range of stretch whilst not straining your muscles.

Walking:

If there was one physical exercise that could be recommended to everyone it would be walking. It is what we are designed for and what activates our entire musculoskeletal system and physiology, as well as being very beneficial to our mental health. Many people find a pedometer that measures the number of steps we take in a day is a valuable aid to ensure we don't neglect this exercise.

The debate continues as to what the optimum number of steps per day is. There isn't a standard number for everyone, it depends on what you are doing when you are not walking, your work, your age, your general health, and your own satisfaction and enjoyment you get from walking. As a rough guide I would suggest a minimum of between 2,000 to 5,000 per day and regard anything over 5,000 as a health bonus!

Postural Improvement:

Staring at our smart phones, computer screens, and sitting at office desks all tend to lead to bad posture. From my own experience, old age can easily cause us to become more stooped if we are not made aware of our posture. If your work involves staring at a computer all day and you normally wear varifocal or bifocal glasses, make sure you get a pair of glasses for your computer work otherwise the constant tilt backwards of your head will generate neck problems for you. Many people also use a raised computer stand to reduce this problem or even stand for some periods at their computer if they can raise it to the right height.

The model of good posture and body use is there for all to see in any two-year-old child, so if you want to learn more about this subject spend a little time studying a two-year-old, how they walk, bend, sit and lift heavy things. Only when we start to make them sit quietly in the wrong seating, at the wrong height of a table or tell them to "stop fidgeting" do they begin to learn our bad habits! I believe the best schools in Sweden adjust the seat and desk heights for their children as they grow!

It is a good mental image to think of an invisible thread lifting us upwards from the top of our head to the heavens, what I call "levity" that balances the other force that keeps us grounded to earth we call "gravity". Levity is light, uplifting and happy, to balance gravity that is heavy, depressing or even sad. Have you noticed how most people when unhappy stoop forward but when happy stand tall and upright? That's my levity and gravity working! The scope and work of physical medicine is beyond this small book, and I would suggest readers might like to gain more insight into this subject by accessing my e-Book "The Body Connection." [15.]

"I have an amazing & miraculous body!"

Chapter 8

The Food Connection

"Let food be thy medicine and medicine be thy food."

Hippocrates 400 BC

Would it make good sense to change your lifestyle and eating habits if all, or most of the following benefits could be gained?

To live a longer healthy and active life, to look and feel younger, to have more energy and vitality, to lose weight if you're overweight, to lower your blood cholesterol, to prevent or reverse heart disease, to lower your risk of developing prostate, breast or other cancers, to preserve your eyesight in later years, to prevent and reverse diabetes, to avoid surgery in many instances, to vastly decrease your need for pharmaceutical drugs, to keep your bones strong, to avoid impotence, to avoid a stroke, to prevent kidney disease, to lower your blood pressure, to reduce the risk of Alzheimer's disease, to beat arthritis and much more.

The results are unmistakable, change your diet and dramatically reduce your risk of cancer, heart disease, diabetes, and obesity! The choice is literally in your hands, or on your knife and fork! [39]

If you believe it would make good sense to check your eating habits considering the above potential benefits, then the question arises how? Traditionally most people wanting to understand and have advice on their diet have needed to consult a professional nutritionist. Where there are complexities in the health of an individual this still may be the best route, but for most of the public there is a very simple and free alternative as described below.

There is a questionnaire called the "4LeafSurvey©" that will give an adequate assessment of the quality of your diet with regards to its impact on your health and disease. The underlying assumption is that for most people, a "Whole Plant Diet" is best for health and for protecting ourselves from disease. For those who want to learn more about the science behind this presumption I would recommend they read a book by Dr. T. Colin Campbell, "The China Study" as a starting point.[17] It was this book that totally changed my understanding of nutrition in health and disease and led me to routinely screen all my patients for dietary quality.

I have always been a lover of simplicity and the "4LeafSurvey©" diet check meets that requirement. Usually when there is a question about diet most people will have several consultations with a nutritionist to establish a detailed analysis of their current diet, to identify any nutritional excesses or deficiencies, and to adjust their diet to help deal with any specific health problems. This approach can be costly and time consuming and often leads to the prescription of many supplements to micro-control the body's digestion and assimilation processes. It has been my experience, that for most people, great benefits can be achieved with the "4LeafSurvey©", and by answering a dozen simple questions in just a few minutes you will have a valuable measure of the quality of your diet and indications as how to improve it.

In essence what this survey does is to give a good estimate of the percentage of your daily calories you get from Whole Plant Foods, which in turn is closely correlated to how your diet is either health promoting or disease risk generating. The way to improve your overall nutrition can then be easily seen from the questionnaire itself. It gives a score that can be from -40 at worst to+ 40 at best, and by repeating the questionnaire as you change your diet you can immediately see whether you are heading in the right direction.

The high negative score is very close to SAD, the Standard American Diet, based on plenty of meat, dairy, refined foods, convenience foods, snacks, fizzy drinks, and creamy rich desserts in large portions, whereas the high positive score is related to a diet which is principally based on vegetables, fruit, pulses, grains, legumes, nuts, seeds, tubers, all unrefined and in great variety. The middle score of -10 to plus +10 is very much the "meat and two veg" variety of diet.

Dietary Information & Guidelines on Whole Plant Nutrition

Note: most people don't need a rapid shift in diet but rather a steady change over weeks makes more sense – *old eating habits are not easy to change!*

The table below gives a very simplified risk assessment of various mixed diets from a typical western mixed animal, dairy, and plant diet (ABD) to a 100% whole plant diet (WPD).

Note: that even a 100% WPD does not guarantee freedom from any health risk, a very small percentage is due to genetics, environmental factors etc. Likewise, a 100% animal-based diet (ABD) does not guarantee development of major disease; just as some people have lived well to 95 years of age smoking 40 a day and heavy drinking, but they are the exception!

The Standard American Diet (SAD) scores -20 to -40.

The UK diet of "meat & two veg" scores (0 to -10)

What is your health risk with your present diet?

The potential risk of such diseases as Alzheimer's Disease, Auto-immune Diseases, Angina, Bowel cancer, Breast cancer, CHD, Diabetes, Hypertension, Liver cancer, Lupus, MS, Stroke, Osteoporosis, Prostate cancer, Rheumatoid arthritis, and many more diseases is closely linked to our diet.

4LeafSurvey Score	Health Risk Associated with Diet
+30 to +40	Minimum risk of chronic disease
+20 to +30	Low risk of chronic disease
+10 to +20	Below average risk of chronic disease
+10 to -10	Average risk of chronic disease
-10 to -20	Above average risk of chronic disease
-20 to -30	High risk of chronic disease
-30 to -40	Maximum risk of chronic disease

A Simple Guide to Healthier Eating Recommendations

Group A Eat all you want (with lots of variety) of any whole, unrefined plant-based foods.

General category	Some examples
Vegetables	Aubergine, artichoke (globe), asparagus, bamboo shoots, broccoli, Brussel sprouts, cauliflower, cabbage, carrots, celery, celeriac, chard, chicory, chillies, coriander, courgettes, cucumber, daikon, endive, garlic, ginger root, green beans, French beans, kale, lettuce, leeks, marrow, mustard cress, okra, olives, onions, peppers, pumpkin, radish, radicchio, secale, shallots, soya, spinach, spring greens, spring onions, squash, Swiss chard, water cress, etc.
Fruit	Apples, apricots, avocado, banana, bilberries, blueberries, blackberries, cherries, cranberries, currants, cucumber, damsons, dates, gooseberries, grapefruit, green pepper, grapes, guavas, kiwi, lemons, limes, loganberries, lychees, mangoes, melon, mandarins, nectarine, pomegranate, quince, raspberries, red currants, rhubarb, strawberries, tangerines, tomato, water melon, white currants, etc.
Starch rich foods	Potatoes, carrots, turnip, beetroot, salsify, swede, parsnips, sweet potatoes, yams, pumpkin, rutabaga, squash, corn on the cob, Jerusalem artichoke, etc.
Pulses & beans	Soya beans, peas, kidney beans, lentils, white beans, peanuts, chickpeas, black beans, adzuki beans, cannellini beans, broad beans, etc.
Mushrooms	White button, cremini, portabella, shitake, oyster, etc.
Dried fruit	Apricots, dates, raisins, apple, figs, currants, prunes, sultanas, etc.
Cereals, grains	Amaranth, arrowroot, barley, buckwheat, bulgar, brown rice, cornmeal, millet, oats, polenta, quinoa, rye, semolina, sorghum, spelt, whole wheat, wild rice, etc.
Nuts, seeds	Walnuts, almonds, macadamia, pecan, cashew, cobnuts, hazelnuts, pistachio, flax seeds, chia seeds, hemp seeds, pumpkin seeds, poppy seeds, tahini, etc.

Group B Minimize the following.

Refined carbohydrates	Pastas (*except whole grain ones*), white bread, crackers, sugars and most cakes, biscuits and pastries made with refined flour and sugar
Vegetable oils	Corn oil, peanut oil, olive oil, etc. (Oil is an extract, not whole plant and see calorific value below for another reason why!)
Fish	Salmon, tuna, cod (*Better than meat but still have "animal food" problems*)

Group C Reduce or avoid where possible.

Meat	Steak, hamburgers, lard, & processed meats(classed as carcinogens by WHO)
Poultry	Chicken, turkey
Dairy	Cheese, milk, yogurt
Eggs	Eggs & egg products with high egg content (e.g. mayonnaise)
Non-food	Sugary, salty snacks full of non food ingredients
Fun drinks	Full of sugar and artificial flavours and colours

Practical advice & help:

1. Try to increase the Group A foods before eliminating Group C foods.
2. Ensure you increase the variety of foods you eat. The simplest and surest way of ensuring you get all the nutrients your body needs is to be constantly adding new foods to your diet.
3. Replace milk with any of the plant-based alternatives; soya, oat, almond, coconut, cashew milk, etc.
4. Try to eliminate dairy first in Group C whilst reducing the portion size of meat, replacing some with fish.
5. You can access the "4LeafSurvey©", to update your score on-line at: <www.4leafsurvey.com> or use the "Quiz" on the Food Connection section on my website <www.TotalHealthMatters.co.uk>
6. Remember, our eating habits have often been with us for decades and to make major changes is a challenge. Those with no major health problems can make small progressive changes over weeks or months, but those people with major health problems should try to effect the change to a Whole Plant Diet as quickly as possible to gain maximum benefit. Note: With no meat or fish in your diet you may need a B12 supplement.
7. One of the problems many people meet when making these changes is "What can we cook now?" Download an excellent App "Forks over Knives" with good recipes or visit: www.pcrm.org/health/diets/recipes

How good is your current diet?

The table below shows the approximate nutritional content of food groups and calories per pound. This table enables you to judge for yourself how nutritionally balanced your current diet is.

Food Group	Vitamins	Calcium mg	Fiber grams	Protein grams	Cholesterol mg	Fat grams	Calories/Pound	Nutrient Density
Vegetables	High	500	30	30	Nil	4	<250	200-1000
Fruits	High	500	30	30	Nil	3	<500	50-200
Potatoes, rice, grains	High	500	30	30	Nil	4	500	30-50
Beans, peas, lentils	Mid	500	50	30	Nil	3	750	50-100
Nuts & seeds	Mid	500	30	30	Nil	6	2500	25-100
Breads	Low	250	30	20	Nil	2	750	10-25
Dried fruits	Mid	500	30	30	Nil	3	1000	25-50
Meat, Fish, Cheeses, Milk, etc.	Minimal	250	Nil	30	140	40	2000	10-20
Dry cereals, popcorn	Low	500	20	30	Nil	2	1500	5-10
Vegetable oils	Nil	Nil	Nil	Nil	Nil	50	4000	2-10
Sugars	Nil	Nil	Nil	Nil	Nil	Nil	1500	1-5

Nutrient content per 500 calories. of Whole Plant Diet & Meat & Dairy Diet . ** Based on Dr. J. Fuhrman's Aggregate Nutrient Density Index

Some Dietary Questions Answered:

Whole Plant Based Diet (WPD) versus a Mixed Dairy and Meat (DMD)

Is there sound evidence that most modern diseases are diet related and that a plant-based diet reduces risk?	Yes! Diabetes, Heart disease, Strokes, Alzheimer's disease, and many Cancers all have strong links to diet.
Does our diet affect our cholesterol levels?	Yes! A PBD lowers it, as it contains no cholesterol. A DMD is the main source of cholesterol in any diet.
Do we need meat to ensure we get adequate protein?	No! Protein content per 100 calories is the same for both diets.
Can we get enough iron from a plant-based diet?	Yes! Ten times more iron in a PBD than DMD
Is it possible to live a healthy life just on plants?	Yes! Only B12 and Vitamin D supplements may be needed for some people.

Do children need dairy produce for growing bones?	No! There is double the calcium content in PBD compared with a DMD.
Can we get vital antioxidants in an animal-based diet?	No! Almost nil in a DMA. PBD is the only significant source for these vital nutrients.
Will we get adequate fiber in an animal-based diet?	No! There is almost no fiber in DMD but high in PBD and essential for our gut health.

More information on the clinical research of Whole Plant Nutrition & Videos by leading doctors on specific health problems can be seen on the website: www.totalhealthmatters.co.uk/food-connection/ or read my eBook "The Food Connection"[51]

CAUTION! Major dietary improvements can usually reduce the need for medications; check with your doctor as you progress with changes in your diet. (Especially diabetics)

To learn more on this subject I would suggest you read my e-Book "The Food Connection"[40] and listen to my podcast "The World's Finest Diet" to be found on Apple Podcasts and other major podcast sites.

"I eat the best foods for my body!"

Chapter 9

The Water Connection

"Water is the driving force of all nature."

Leonado da Vinci (1452-1519)

"You are not sick, you are thirsty."

Dr. F. Batmanghelidj

Water is a unique fluid that we are only just beginning to understand. It is the main substance of our bodies, it is what makes our planet the dynamic, flourishing, amazing biosphere bursting with life forms. Yet most of us are almost unaware of the importance of our water consumption for healthy living.

We can survive weeks without food but only a few days without water, we are 75% made of water, we don't have copper wires to carry nerve signals, our nerves are fluid wires, and our brain is 85% water. Imagine the consequences of serious water loss, how it would affect the entire functioning of our body and in particular our nervous system and our ability to use our brain.

Besides this water is a unique fluid with many strange properties we are now only beginning to understand, so it is no use thinking you can replace pure water with any other fluid or beverage to meet the body's demand for water. It doesn't work. Most of our chosen drinks like tea, coffee, beer, wine, fizzy drinks not only don't add to the body's water supply but usually cause increased elimination of water so that we lose more than we take in.

Most of us would say, don't worry because we know when we need water, we get thirsty and have a dry mouth. Sadly, this is not true, the thirst for water and a dry mouth is at the extreme end of water shortage while the body has been suffering dehydration for some time.

So, what does water do for our bodies? The greatest authority on this subject is Doctor Batmanghelidj who spent a lifetime of research studying the role of water in our lives. In his book "You're not sick, you're thirsty! [16] He lists forty-six reasons why your body needs water every day. I will give just a few of these reasons here; there is no life without water, water is the prime solvent for all foods, water is the transport system of nutrients for the body, water clears toxins from the body, water lubricates our joints, water is the essential fluid for our cooling system-sweating, adequate water protects our blood from clotting while circulating and water is involved in all energy exchange systems in the body.

Dehydration is almost an epidemic today laying the foundation for many common ailments from asthma and allergies to stress and strokes. It appears as we age, we become less sensitive to the need for water and many elderly people are often severely dehydrated.

So, summarizing some of the Myths in medicine about water:

• A dry mouth is the only sign of dehydration. The truth is a dry mouth is the very last sign of dehydration.
• Water is a simple liquid. Water is now recognized as a remarkable unique liquid crystal fluid: it is life-sustaining and health-promoting.
• The body can regulate water needs and intake. Our perception of thirst is not reliable: as we get older it fails us.
• Any fluid can replace water. Most other fluids: tea, coffee, fizzy drinks, alcohol, etc. not only do not replace water but may cause loss of water. Every day the body becomes short of 6 to 10 glasses of water.

Advice:
Drink water before eating.
Always drink water when thirsty even during a meal.
Drink water 2 to 3 hours after a meal.
Drink water first thing in the morning to correct for loss during sleep.

Drink water before exercising, to prepare for sweating.
Drink more water if constipated; 2 to 3 glasses in the morning act as a good laxative.
So just how much water do we need to protect ourselves from the ravages of dehydration?

Your Guide to How Much Water You Need:

Your weight in pounds	Your weight in kilos.	Ideal Water Intake Fluid oz.	Ideal Water Intake litres	Glasses (8 fl.oz) of Water
8 to 100	35 to 45	40 to 50	1 to 1.5	5 to 6
100 to 150	45 to 70	50 to 75	1.5 to 2	6 to 9
150 to 200	70 to 90	75 to 100	2 to 3	9 to 12
200 to 250	90 to 115	100 to 125	3 to 3.5	12 to 15

Water Deserves Far More Attention

At times discoveries can shake our perception of the world and our lives. A book written by Masaru Emoto, "The Hidden Messages in Water" [25] should have this impact on all those reading it. His research began with the observation that no two ice crystals are the same! His belief that water could hold information then led him to develop a method of recording this. What better way than to freeze water and photograph the resulting crystal forms. Would there be patterns that distinctly varied with information input? His book is a record of this research with actual photographs of water subjected to varying forms of information.

He has produced water crystals after music has been played close to it, where the quality of the crystals changed with the quality of the music, after children have spoken repeatedly to it, either kindly or rudely and after words have been written on the bottle containing the water. The forms and complexity reflected the information input almost without exception.

This should not have been a surprise to me, as for most of my career I have accepted the validity of homoeopathy (unlike the general medical profession) and how the "image" of any remedy is established in water and then has specific actions on the patient, *even when there is no material presence of the original substance, but only the image of the substance.* Yet, because of the institutional objection to this hypothesized effect, I like others, had not fully embraced the significance of this concept. It takes time to re-educate oneself, to undo the indoctrination of "old flat earth thinkers"!

Dr. Emoto has met with Dr. Rupert Sheldrake and together their research work is complimenting each other's. The Morphic Resonance [41] fields proposed by Dr. Sheldrake are being visually confirmed with Dr. Emoto's water crystallization. He goes on to say:

"The important thing about Dr. Sheldrake's theory is that once the morphic resonance has spread, it extends to all space and all time. In other words, if a morphic field is formed, it will have an instantaneous impact on all other locations, resulting in an instantaneous worldwide change. When I first heard about Dr. Sheldrake's theory, I couldn't contain my interest, because my research into water crystals was nothing less than an attempt to express the resonance of the morphic field in a way that can be seen with the naked eye." [24]

Dr. Emoto discusses universal consciousness and the view that each of us reflects this:

"In my opinion, a doctor who treats the human body must first be a philosopher. In the past, the doctor was the community shaman or priest, exhorting people to follow the laws of nature, live their lives correctly, and make use of the healing powers found in nature.

If doctors were to treat not only the sick parts of the body but also the human consciousness, then I think we would see a great reduction in the need for doctors and hospitals. People with ailments would go to their nearby philosopher, for help in understanding the mistakes they had made, and then go home determined to live a better life. It may well be that the physicians of the future will be more like councilors than the doctors we have today.

I have talked with many people about their health problems and have come to see that ailments are largely a result of negative emotions. If you can erase such emotions, you have an innate capacity to recover from illness. The importance of being positive cannot be under-estimated. Positive thinking will strengthen your immune system and help you set you moving towards recovery, a fact that the medical community is starting to wake up to.

For instance, there is a doctor who treats his cancer patients with mountain climbing. Giving people a reason to live boosts their spirits and their immune system.

There's also an increase in interest in holistic medicine not only treating the symptoms of the illness but overseeing the patient's lifestyle and psychological well-being. In fact, doctors have recently formed an organization called the Japan Holistic Medical Society, to promote this type of medicine in Japan. The days of believing only that which can be seen by the naked eye have passed, and we are now starting to open our eyes to the importance of the soul. It's a move in the right direction, and I think it will become the way the majority think within this century.

The human body is essentially water, and consciousness is the soul. Methods to help water to flow smoothly are superior to all other medical methods available to us. It's all about keeping the soul in an unpolluted state. Can you imagine what it would be like to have water capable of forming beautiful crystals flowing throughout your entire body, it can happen if you let it. Among all medicines there are none with the healing powers of love, since I came to this realization, I have continued to tell people that immunity is love what could be more effective at overcoming negative powers and returning vitality to the body? However I have recently felt the need to change my terminology fully, I now know that it is not love alone that forms immunity but love and gratitude. ...." [25]

"I drink all the water I need!"

Chapter 10

The Breath Connection

"The perfect man breathes as though he is not breathing."

Lao Tzu circa 4th century BC.

"The more you breathe the nearer you are to death, the less you breathe the longer your life."

Prof. Konstantin Buteyko (1923-2003)

It has taken me my whole career working as a therapist to eventually recognise the proverbial elephant in the healthcare room. It is curious too, that the animal of this proverb is the elephant, as the elephant is long lived, has an amazing nose for breathing, has remarkable teeth that formed the tusks, lives entirely on plant food and lives in a close family community. All these elements of this animal have a bearing about the breath connection.

It would be difficult to argue that breathing is not the most important activity in our lives; we can live without food for three weeks, without water for three days but without breathing for a mere three minutes. We arrive in this world with our first breath and a cry, take about half a billion breaths during our stay and leave with a sigh. However modern medicine shows little interest in breathing unless we present with some serious pathology that affects it, and generally your doctor won't check your breathing should you visit for a health check.

The elephant, like all mammals, including you and I, has the allotted half billion breaths, but he breathes quietly and slowly and often attains a ripe old age of over a hundred in good health. He, like all mammals, habitually breathes through his nose that further ensures a long healthy life as we shall see later. Although he may have remarkably overgrown teeth as tusks, he, like all other mammals, won't need orthodontic work for crooked or crowded teeth, his wholly plant-based diet aids his health and finally his close family group provides the ideal support during the early years and in old age.

Another interesting thing about breathing is that we don't all eat from the same plate or drink from the same cup, but *we all share the same air when we breathe*. Surely breathing is the most sociable thing we do, when we take a breath of air in, we will be inhaling a little of the exhaled air of every living person and animal on the planet!

Now that's quite a breath connection if ever there was!

I suppose it is because we never need to think about our breathing, as it is a wholly automatic and mainly unconscious activity, that we naturally give it little or no attention. We may be more concerned about what we drink and eat since we know we can get this so badly wrong that it can make us ill, but I'm sure most of us don't even consider it matters how much or how we breathe or so long as we do! Yes, we do breathe to stay alive, but the function of breathing is primarily to ensure every cell in the body is oxygenated adequately. It is not about getting air in and out of the lungs as much as possible to have plenty of oxygen, as we live in a "sea of oxygen", as 20% of the air we breathe in and 16% of the air we breathe out is oxygen. If this were not so, it would not be lifesaving to give mouth to mouth resuscitation to provide oxygen to someone who has stopped breathing.

Carbon dioxide, far from being a waste gas could be regarded as the hormone par excellence, that is responsible for the functioning of almost all our body's chemistry. There is no living thing on the planet that can survive without carbon dioxide. A good illustration of this fact is when we marvel at some great oak tree of hundreds of years old and remember it's made mostly of carbon dioxide and water! The breaths from the sheep and the shepherds over those years and the other animals supplied a large part of its food for growth. There is no life as we know it without carbon dioxide. When we digest our food and expend energy we generate large quantities of carbon dioxide, and it is also true that we need to remove excess carbon dioxide, but far from being a waste gas, carbon dioxide is vital for all life. We would not survive without it, in fact it's prime importance for our survival is demonstrated by the fact that our breathing rate is not governed by the level of oxygen in our body, but by the level of carbon dioxide. So, carbon dioxide is not the nasty, lethal gas we have been led to believe but the very foundation of our life.

My experience of over forty years treating patients and checking their breathing, is that over 75% breathe badly and that this fact contributes to their health problems either principally or to a significant extent. Most of us in the West suffer from Chronic Hidden Hyperventilation (CHHV) that has become a hidden or ignored epidemic.[5] Professor Buteyko claimed that over one hundred diseases are associated with or caused by CHHV, including: asthma, angina, anxiety, allergies, digestive problems, gastric reflux, hay fever, heart problems, high blood pressure, hypoxia, IBS, insomnia, snoring, low energy, to mention just a few.

You may wonder how good is your own breathing?

The simplest way of checking this for yourself is to measure your "Control Pause". The Control Pause was the main measure of breathing quality developed by Professor Konstantin Buteyko as part of his breath training programme, now referred to as the Buteyko Method.

To measure your Control Pause you will need some form of timer, a stopwatch, your smart phone, or use the video timer.[45]

1. Sit quietly and relax for a few minutes to establish your normal breathing pattern at rest.
2. Keep your mouth closed all through the test, only breathing through your nose.
3. Take a full breath in through your nose, and when you breathe out, start your timer or stopwatch.
4. You may gently hold your nose to ensure you don't accidently breathe in at this stage.
5. When you feel you need to breathe in remove your nose-hold and check the timer.
6. The number of seconds you were able to hold your breath comfortably is a measure of your control pause.

This breath hold should not be stressful or forced.

The table below gives the evaluation of your control pause:

Control Pause	CO2	Your Breathing State
45-60 seconds	5 - 6 %	Excellent normal breathing.
35-45 seconds	4.5 – 5%	Good but slight over-breathing
25-35 seconds	4 - 4.5%	Moderate hyperventilation
20-25 seconds	3.5 – 4%	High hyperventilation affecting your health
15-20 seconds	3 - 3.5%	Serious hyperventilation
10-15 seconds	2.5 – 3%	Severe hyperventilation
< 10 seconds	< 2.5%	Critically poor breathing

If you have a Control Pause of under 30 seconds you may want to begin training yourself to improve your breathing. The notes below will give you the outline of how to go about this, but you might prefer more formal training. This could be with a Buteyko Educator face to face, an online training course, a podcast training course or you may want to start with just a book on this subject. The Buteyko Guide to Better Breathing & Better Health by Michael Lingard (This book complements my Buteyko Method training podcast) [18].

The Basics of Better Breathing & Better Health

The first step is learning the fact that ***most of us suffer some degree of CHHV*** or chronic hidden hyperventilation, over-breathing in simple terms. Secondly ***CHHV makes us ill!*** Anything from low energy, poor sleep to serious health problems such as asthma, hypertension, sleep apnoea or panic attacks.

Most of us arrived at this state because of the many stressful events in our lives, emotional, physical, illnesses, chemical or whatever. Any stress triggers a primitive response called the "Fight or Flight Syndrome" that once protected us from sabre toothed tigers but today is not so useful and more often has an adverse effect on our health. The Fight or Flight response produces over a thousand physiological changes in our bodies preparing us for emergency action, all but three of these responses we have little or no control over, e.g. histamine production, adrenaline production, corticosteroid production etc.

We can however take conscious control over three of them, our muscle tension, our breathing, and our mental tension. The neat thing is that **once we start to take control over muscle tension, mental tension, and our breathing all the others are reduced.**

There is a very detailed physiological explanation for the benefits of better breathing that you can learn about later. Right now, all you need to know is that CHHV causes us to lose carbon dioxide (carbon dioxide, far from being the deadly gas many of us have been led to believe, is the essential stuff of all living things, we would be dead without it! We need around 6% in our bodies to function well)

Carbon dioxide is so important to our life that **our breathing is governed by the level of carbon dioxide in our blood, and not by the level of oxygen**. Receptors in the brain measure the level of carbon dioxide and adjust our breathing accordingly, if too much we are made to breathe more to "wash out" the excess, if too low we are made to breathe less to conserve it.

With CHHV our receptors have been set at too low a level of carbon dioxide and much of the breath training will be to correct this returning them to normal.

Low carbon dioxide levels cause:

a) Spasm of smooth muscle wrapped around all hollow organs in our body, blood vessels, airways, bladder, gut, etc.

b) The blood's ability to deliver oxygen to all our tissues is impaired and

c) the pH, or acid/alkalinity of the body, is changed affecting every chemical reaction in our bodies adversely.

There are many other effects associated with poor breathing, you can learn about later.

So, how do you correct your breathing if you need to? *First you need a measure of your breathing*. This is based on *two very simple checks you can do yourself, namely, the "control pause" and "pulse" measurements*. The control pause (CP) is a measure of your maximum

COMFORTABLE breath hold, in seconds, after a normal exhalation and, while at rest. Effectively it measures how well your body is oxygenated, if you're well oxygenated you don't need another breath for a sometime, if very poorly oxygenated you will want to take the next breath almost immediately. The Pulse is measured on your wrist or neck by counting the number of beats in 15 seconds and multiplying by four to give number of beats per minute.

Before you start re-training your breathing, please note that breathing has a powerful effect on our entire body and therefore, any exercises should be done with caution. If you have a history of any serious condition including diabetes, heart disease, hypertension, psychotic conditions, severe asthma, etc. you are advised to only do breath training with the support and supervision of your doctor, health professional or Buteyko Educator. This also applies to *anyone* with a CP of under 15 seconds.

Now you can begin:

Try to **always breathe through your nose**, breathing in *and out* through it. If you have a stuffy or blocked nose you will need to clear it with this simple exercise: take a breath in, then out and gently hold your nose while nodding ten times keeping your mouth closed. Release your nose and breathe in through your nose. Repeat as necessary. Check how you are breathing; hold one hand on your chest and the other on your belly, which hand is being moved the most? Try to get all the movement low down where your diaphragm is.

Now you can *measure your CP and pulse with a stopwatch or other timer such as your smart phone or wristwatch.*

When you are *sitting relaxed*, take a good breath in and then out, start your timing and gently hold your nose.

When you feel the need to breathe in, release your nose, take a breath in, and note how long you held your breath for. (Your breath hold should be your *maximum comfortable breath hold* and should not be stressful.) This is your Control Pause measure.

To measure your pulse, find your pulse on your wrist or on your neck, count how many beats you feel in 15 seconds then multiply by four to give your pulse rate in beats per minute.

Now practice **Relaxed or Reduced breathing. Start by simply relaxing, do not try to reduce your breathing at this stage.**
- a) Relax every muscle in your body, be "soft like a cloth!"
- b) Only breathe through the nose, keep your mouth shut.
- c) Try to keep the daily mental stresses out of your mind by occupying your mind with something calming like imagining a garden, seashore, or desert island.
- d) Sit upright with a straight back and both legs placed on the floor.
- e) Close your eyes.
- f) Sit like this, just learning to relax thoroughly for two to five minutes then open your eyes and wait for another minute while resting, to let your breathing return to its new normal.
- g) **Now measure your CP and pulse again.**
- h) If you have succeeded in doing this exercise well, your CP will be higher, and your pulse may be lower or the same. This will mean you are breathing less.
- i) **That was your first exercise in resetting your carbon dioxide receptors.**

Repeat this exercise three or four times a day and keep a record of your results to measure your progress. Alternatively, you can start a formal re-training course with a Buteyko Educator, or with the aid of my podcast training course and an accompanying book to record your progress.[18]

"My breathing is perfect!"

Chapter 11

The Mind Connection

"You are your thoughts and beliefs."

Anon

"Your beliefs become your thoughts, your thoughts become your words, your words become your actions, your actions become your habits, your habits become your value, your value has become your destiny."

Mahatma Gandhi (1869-1948)

The most amazing new knowledge about the human brain is that it has the ability to grow, change, re-arrange all our thoughts and mental processes from birth to death. We have a "plastic" brain that can do remarkable things such as cope with and reorganise all the activities that were done in one area that is now damaged and learn to do them in another area. Areas of the brain that are normally associated with speech can be used for sight or hearing. The old thinking was that we were born with a brain divided up into little boxes and each were allocated a specific job, this has all changed with the latest research.

The greatest error in modern medicine may be the dismissal as trivial the so called "Placebo Effect". Tomorrow's medicine will, I sincerely hope, begin to amend its ways, and give the respect and understanding to this potent force in our lives. Even now, research is demonstrating that the beneficial effect of many medicines may be anything from just a few percent to almost 100 percent due to the placebo effect. There is also the placebo effect's partner, the Nocebo Effect, which is just as powerful in affecting us adversely, just as the Placebo Effect affects us beneficially.

So, what is the mind? It would be a brave or foolhardy man who thought he could give a definition of this. It is almost as undefinable as health, as discussed earlier. We all have an intuitive understanding of what both words mean but perhaps they are concepts too large to be suitable for simple definition.

What we may all agree on is that our mind somehow powerfully influences our body and our actions all the time. Is our mind the same as our brain? Well, there must be some close association because it is only with the aid of our brain can we think and perform all our daily activities of walking, talking, seeing etc.

The best insight I have found so far is that we may consider the brain operating as two halves. We have a conscious brain that allows us to think, plan, remember and express ourselves in our actions and behaviour, and a sub-conscious brain that takes care of all the routine activities that keep us alive and working, our walking, driving the car, cleaning our teeth, digesting our meals, healing our wounds etc.

Here comes the shock for many people, as it was for me, our conscious brain, although it can look into the future and plan, remember events in the past and allow us to be thoughtful and analytical and imaginative in wonderful ways, it can only process about 40 bits of information per second. Whereas our sub-conscious brain, our hidden and usually unrecognized brain can process over 20 million bits of information per second. The major question for all of us is which part of these two brains governs our lives? The answer is that a mere 5% of our behaviour and conscious activity is governed by the conscious brain, and that 95% of our behaviour and activity is governed by the unconscious or sub-conscious brain! Until I learned this, I really thought I was a rational, intelligent individual who was in full charge of my own life! I now realize that is not true and that my sub-conscious mind is the major driving force, but I don't know what it's up to! Is it helping or hindering me to live a full and optimal life, or is it secretly sabotaging my conscious finest endeavours?

What information does our sub-conscious brain have? Does it have negative, painful, memories? Does have uplifting happy memories? Do these memories affect all our actions and behaviour in our lives? We now believe that most of the information held in the sub-conscious brain was laid down before we were seven years old and has been added to over the years when we are going through strong emotional periods, good or bad. Few of us can recall much about our earliest childhood events that lay hidden. Was it the strict father who repeatedly told you that you were a bad child, or the early teacher who called you stupid, or the nanny who kept calling you a lazy good-for-nothing child that are still affecting your life today? For most of us the answer will be "Yes!" Perhaps this explains why you lack confidence, or feel you must work extremely hard to prove you are not lazy, or why you don't think much about yourself or even don't love yourself much? Some of our sub-conscious programme may be added beyond seven years old. I recall a mild caning by the headmaster at a private school for telling a lie when I was ten years old. My children find it amusing that even decades on I find it difficult to tell even the smallest "white lie". Perhaps any traumatic event in adulthood can be added to our store of sub-conscious experiences and further change our behaviour and life without our knowing.

Wouldn't it be great if we could sift through all the bad sub-conscious information and replace it with better, more life enhancing information? Rather like replacing an out-of-date programme with the latest upgrade in your computer hard drive.

Until recently many have worked hard to do just this with the aid of hypnosis, psychotherapy, NLP, positive-thinking, and counselling with varying degrees of success, and usually over a long period of time and with great determination. Having read the work of a few radical thinkers I discovered PSYCH-K [46] and attended a short three-day introductory course on this technique. I have been impressed by two aspects of this therapy. This is only one of several similar systems, the general impact of our two-brain mind is best described in a video by Bruce Lipton.[48] The first is that it recognises that *you are the best authority* on who you are and what you want. *Who knows you better than yourself? Who has nurtured you from birth? Who can change your lifestyle but you? Who but you can change your actions?* This therapy *is not done to you,* but it *is done with you*, with your consent and in your own way. The PSYCH-K practitioner is *a facilitator* and not a therapist in the usual way of

58

thinking. The second aspect of this approach is that rather than hours or weeks of consultations and therapy, you usually "re-programme your hard drive" or change your sub-conscious content yourself in minutes. The founder of this system is Rob Williams who defines PSYCH-K as:

"A non-invasive, interactive process of change with a proven record of success for over 25 years. A simple yet powerful process to change subconscious beliefs that are self-limiting and self-sabotaging. A unique blend of various tools for change, some contemporary and some ancient, derived from contemporary neuroscience research, as well as ancient mind/body wisdom. A groundbreaking approach to facilitating change at the subconscious level where at least 95% of our consciousness operates. A process that transcends the standard method of visualization, affirmations, will power, and positive thinking, especially effective in areas of behaviour/habit change, wellness, and stress reduction."

This does not in any way suggest that all other therapeutic systems are not effective and successful for most people, but PSYCH-K opens yet another potential route that may appeal to those who want to try to be their own healers as much as possible. This has been the key challenge of medicine and healthcare throughout the ages; finding the right therapy and support for the individual that is best suited at that time and stage in their life. At the simplest level it makes sense not to "beat ourselves up" when we perform badly or make a mistake, and it is well known that repetition is a slow but effective way of reprogramming our sub-conscious data store. There is an old saying used by actors "fake it, until you make it!". If you are not well, repeat to yourself "I am well" whenever you remember, it may be a lie, but you can fool your sub-conscious mind!

If there is just one mind problem that deserves most attention in today's world it is very simply "Stress". The World Health Organization has recently stated that stress is the leading cause of early mortality. The explanation for this is that stress from whatever source triggers our primitive survival response of "fight/flight" or "fight/flight/freeze". As an evolutionary survival mechanism, it has enabled man to cope with everything from attacks from sabre tooth tigers, violent weather conditions, threats from aggressive neighbours to modern day work and living stressors. Unfortunately, repeated frequent stressors create the health hazard when there are no periods between stressors to recover normal physiology and damage repair to our bodies.

Luckily, once again, we can learn to take control of our reaction to life's stressors, by improving our "response-ability", which is the common message throughout this journey of becoming "Your Own Doctor of Health & Happiness". By improving our breathing quality, it is the most direct way of minimising the impact of stress. It is almost impossible to be stressed when we are breathing in a slow, gentle way.

" I am strong, healthy, and happy!"

Chapter 12

The Family & Community Connection

The Peckham Experiment

"Our separation from each other is an optical illusion of consciousness".

Albert Einstein (1879-1955)

"We are creating a habitat that diverges more and more and
with increasing speed from that to which genetic evolution has adapted us."

Niko Tinbergen, Nobel Prize winner (1907-1988)

As part of my passion to discover the fundamentals of health and well-being I studied the work of a remarkable doctor, Dr. Scott-Williamson. In his later years, as a brilliant pathologist, he asked himself a very simple question that would become the basis for his work and research for the rest of his life. As a pathologist he was reasonably happy that he knew the aetiology of most common diseases, what were the key causes of each disease, that was his profession, but when he asked himself, what was the aetiology of health, what in other words were the key causes of health, he had no answer.

He then began a search through all published research papers in this country and abroad but could find little on the subject. What he knew, as most of us would agree, is that health isn't just what's left after we remove all diseases, it is far more than that.

To summarise over twenty years research, in just a few words, what he discovered was that health was based on a child growing up with a father and mother in a community that supports them as a family. He also took for granted that the child needed an adequate diet, exercise, and an environment where he or she could develop his or her own talents as fully as possible.

This conclusion was based on the experience of over a thousand families who were part of what became called the Peckham Experiment.

In Peckham, in London, a large modern building was designed with swimming pool, gymnasium, cafeteria, creche, and areas for outdoor recreations, as well as a medical unit where all participating families had their annual health audit. Anyone who was found in need of medical attention or further tests was advised to see their own doctor, whether they did or not was their decision. This was all part of encouraging self-responsibility for their own health and that of their family.

By every medical measure, the health of all participants improved year on year. It was regarded as the most important medical research of its time and the centre had thousands of visitors from home and abroad every year, including the Queen.

When the NHS was being planned by Aneurin Bevin, a group approached the government to propose that similar centres should be established throughout the country to improve the health and well-being of the nation. The other group that approached the government suggested that if people had better access to modern medicine this would ensure a healthier nation. We now know who won the day, and only now are we seeing a growing recognition that drugs and medical interventions do not always lead to improved health and cure of the disease, but usually they simply help manage disease and ameliorate symptoms.

If Dr. Scott-Williamson was right, that our own health and the health of our nation is built on family and community, it may explain why there is so much sickness in the UK. As a nation, we may lead the world in this, as we have a record of ever-increasing numbers of broken families and poor community support, those two prime factors that Dr. Scott-Williamson and his co-worker Dr. Innes-Pearce, proved were essential for the development of a healthy child.

We are seeing a worrying rise in childhood mental problems through stress and anxiety, not helped by social media and the growing preference of connecting with our smart phones rather than our friends, besides the adverse effects of diet and lack of exercise leading to an epidemic of obesity and related diseases.

The very word health is derived from Hale, old English for whole. The rationale behind the Peckham experiment findings is that for a child to fully develop as a whole person they need a secure environment of a mother and father, as only when we have the union of male and female is there a whole human. Every man is essentially half a human as is every woman but together they represent a model of a whole human that the child learns from.

The rich environment of many families meeting, working, eating, and playing together in the Peckham Centre increased the possibility of children growing to their fullest potential.

All the latest research is pointing to the importance of our childhood development from birth to early schooling, and how this experience can strengthen or weaken the child for life. As another pioneer in this area Dr. Glenn Doman says, "education begins at around six years of age, but our learning begins at birth". In fact, the capacity of a toddler to learn is many thousands of times greater than an adult's learning ability. Dr. Glenn Doman also asserted that *every child born has a greater potential intelligence than Leonardo da Vinci ever had, with no exceptions!* Remember the fact mentioned in the mind section that the sub-conscious mind can process information millions of times faster than our conscious mind and this occurs naturally in a child under seven. It explains why a child brought up in a family where two or more languages are spoken learns fluency in them all without effort! This should make us all rethink our view of the tiny baby and toddler as not being as simple a creature as we have been led to believe, but to recognise the fact that we are nurturing a potential genius with a greater capacity to learn than we ever thought possible.

Whilst reviewing literature I have read over the years for this book I came upon a most powerful book called "Being Me and Also Us, Lessons from the Peckham Experiment" by Alison Stallibrass. In this book a detailed description of the workings of the Peckham Experiment is given as well as the conclusions derived from the experiment. I believe it is essential reading for all those interested in health of our society in the future.[23]

Let me quote from this book:

"That health is something positive, something more than the absence of disease and disability has always been instinctively known: the 'blooming cheek', 'clear eye', 'shining hair' or 'springing step'. Now, nearly half a century after Peckham Biologists demonstrated this truth in an experimental situation and tried to make it accepted as a fact by the established leaders of thought and makers of policy, it is at last seeping into people's conscious thoughts, and they are beginning to ponder its implications.

An understanding and acceptance of the idea, put forward by the Peckham Biologists, that health is basically a *process of realizing one's potential for maturity* would make communication about health easier and the practice of education healthier.

If health is a process of mutual subjective synthesis of organism and environment and person and group, it is not something that members of the medical profession can give us. They can only remove or alleviate the pathological conditions that prevent us from engaging in the process of health. *The responsibility for a person's health lies firstly with himself* and, secondly, with anyone who has any power to influence his environment, lawmakers, administrators, planners, architects, teachers, farmers, processes of food stuffs and parents.

Therefore, I believe that people will have to make up their own minds individually what they want in a way of means of cultivating health, find out how it may be obtained, and go out and get it for themselves.

As I have suggested, it is probably the parents of young children more than any other class of people who are strongly moved to create for themselves an environment in which health may be cultivated. It seems to me that many of them feel that the purpose of life is life, and the prime responsibility is to the next generation. And some have a similar confidence to that which developed in the Peckham Centre, in the capacity for spontaneous growth of every living being, and a person's inborn urge to grow, and in his power to recognize the nourishment that his faculties and abilities need at any moment in order to grow, as long as his environment contains suitable opportunities for nourishment. Many among them also know that does not help children to have parents who feel they must sacrifice their own growth for their children's sake. They know as the Peckham Biologists knew that the best surroundings for a child are such as contained people who are rejoicing in their own growth and who enjoy doing whatever they're doing at the moment (including the household chores and whatever else is necessary for the creation of a home that gives pleasure and allows the family individuality to develop)." pages 254-255.[23]

"I am grateful to all my family and community!"

Chapter 13

The Environmental Connection

"The medical assumption is that war against disease gives rise to health. However, health in the individual, the family, and occasionally in the community establishes itself without any medical intervention........"

"Recognising Health" by Kenneth Barlow [53]

This is almost an echo of an early discussion of the prime importance of environment on our genetic activity. It is now accepted that our genes are switched on or off by signals from our environment whether that be internal or external. The internal environment includes the subtle thoughts we have to the biochemical changes in our blood and the processes of digestion. The external environment includes our immediate physical surroundings: our housing, garden, street, the air we breathe, the water we are supplied with, the plants and animals around us, our workplace, the community, and the entire planet.

If we accept the fact that we are immersed in and connected with the total environment from inner to outer, it would be reasonable to suggest our individual health and wellbeing is derived from this entire complex of connections, some have more profound impact than others, but it appears we are far more than we ever believed. *Are you a reflection of the Universe?*

This concept requires a paradigm shift in our normal thinking. We are very much like our ancestors whom we now regard as rather "unintelligent or simple minded" because they believed the earth was flat. We have slowly acquired an arrogant attitude that modern man is far superior, more scientific, and rational, but have we really changed that much? I think humanity needs more humility to recognise its advances yet be open to the infinite dimension of what we need still to learn. I like a simple mind experiment I have given to some of my patients on this topic, "visualize that all the information about everything in the universe we shall ever know, fills the room you are standing in, how much do we know already? Is it most of the room, half the room, a substantial chunk of the room or do you think it is little more than a cupful or even a teaspoonful?" Most people I have asked tended to choose a cupful or less. *Maybe this is because of our innate wisdom?*

This common barrier to advancing our understanding of life and the universe was seen by Leonardo da Vinci (1452-1519), whose exceptional significance and reputation was not only due to his brilliant talents in art, but also because he was an exceptional scientist. Dr. T. Colin Campbell wrote in his book 'Whole" [42] that da Vinci's contributions to our understanding of the universe were so profound and enduring precisely because of this integration. He realised holism needed reductionism to advance and reductionism needed holism to remain relevant. He realised that when you take something out of context to study it more closely or measure it exactly you risk losing more wisdom than you gain. This same criticism is echoed in the book, "The Science Delusion" Freeing the Spirit of Enquiry, by Rupert Sheldrake [43].

We might be witnessing morphic resonance, the brainchild of Rupert Sheldrake and others, gaining strength, or is it simply my being on the look-out for it? I recently read an article about the greater power of positive parenting as opposed to "good old fashioned childhood training enforced with the naughty step", in a book "There's No Such Thing as Naughty" by Kate Silverton, and then I listened to the groundbreaking establishment of a school to rehabilitate young offenders called Oasis Reform, a secure school with no bars, no cells, no warders, but designed to provide real support to young offenders who have been emotionally traumatised by not having had a good start in life. As the speaker said, "why should we have our physical traumas treated with healing work in a hospital, but our mental traumas merit us being punished in a prison? "Is there a new growing awareness of a better way for mankind fuelled not with hate, greed, and fear, with the resulting wars and individual suffering, but nurtured with love, gratitude, and courage that leads to healing and happiness? I believe so!

" I am helping form a better environment!"

Chapter 14

The Earth Connection

Healthy individual, healthy family, healthy society, healthy earth.

Anon.

It is impossible to discuss the health and well-being of an individual in any complete way without studying the impact of the whole environment upon them. I have discussed this in relation to our genes, that it is now accepted that our genes are turned on or turned off by the environment around, that is both internal environment of our bloodstream and the external environment we live in both physically and socially.

This may seem a distant and almost irrelevant connection when viewed from our personal experience, but we must remember we all live on the same biosphere we call earth. The places we live and work impact on our health through the body connection, the earth, soil, oceans, and water affect the food we eat through the food connection, the air we breathe affects our health through the breath connection, the social and economic stresses of our interconnected world may impact on our mental health through the mind connection, and our close friends family and community have a profound impact on our health through the living connection. So, it would be reasonable to assume the health and sustainability of the global environment should play a vital part in the health and well-being of every individual.

The environmental damage from pollution, overconsumption, and the destruction of habitat and forests, has been well documented and understood by most of us now. The universal problem appears just too large to attempt a solution, particularly for the individual, but it is a problem that could be solved by millions of individuals if we all worked in the right direction to solve it. This is probably beyond the capacity of any government but not beyond the capacity of mankind.

A few years ago, I published an article for a health magazine that was based on the old tradition of establishing New Year's resolutions. It outlined the twelve steps we can all take over twelve months that would have a significant impact on the health of our planet. It seems appropriate that I repeat this here if we are to effect the dramatic changes we must make.

A Challenge to Improve Our Health and the Health of Our Planet

If everyone on the Internet joined forces to ensure a healthy planet for future generations, it could solve our survival problems that no government dare tackle. All you need to do is commit to a changing lifestyle over 12 months - a twelve step programme just a month at a time. Check the references for tips. No need to start in January as a New Year Resolution but start right now whatever the month!

January: try to avoid buying anything made of or packed in plastic. Plastics are based on fossil fuel for production and produce an almost permanent environmental pollutant that will take hundreds of years to start to rectify. There are bio-degradable alternative materials produced from plants. [26]

February: buy local produce wherever possible. This would both stimulate farmers to shift to plant food production for humans, reduce the vast energy consumption involved in shipping food to and from warehouses and from abroad.[27]

March: We need cut back on our consumption of "stuff". We are all encouraged to consume or buy far more material things than we really need, we must remind ourselves that every article represents a substantial use of the earth's scarce resources.[28]

April: help plant 100 trees with the estimated 4 billion internet users worldwide. This would produce 400 billion trees, the most efficient carbon dioxide consumers, would remove around 8 billion tons of CO2 per year, that would help balance the residual fossil fuel use. Global production of CO2 from transport is about this same quantity. [29]

May: support your local community any way that helps the environment. There is a close connection between the health of the planet, the health of individuals, and the health of a community. By building stronger communities we would find mutual support in building a sustainable future for our only planet, the earth. [30]

June: cut out all meat, fish, and dairy foods from your diet. This alone would cut greenhouse gases by between 25 to 50%, stop the loss of the earth's lungs - the rainforests, reduce the need for food production by 75%, and with the right distribution system ensure adequate food for everyone, improve the health of everyone, reduce the incidence of chronic disease, reduce the pollution of coastal waters from agricultural and medical run-off and animal waste, permit the regrowth of our fauna and flora, especially endangered species, and much more. Currently estimates suggest between 50 to 75% of all grain and pulses go to feed animals![31]

July: Conserve freshwater wherever possible. It is a scarce resource and will become even scarcer in the future and more valuable than oil. Sources of fresh water are increasingly being depleted due to pollution or overexploitation. Producing animal and dairy foods is a major reason for this.[32]

August: make your own health your responsibility. This is very much the theme of the book you are now reading. If you have already shifted your diet to a whole plant-based diet and are getting more exercise walking, you're well on the way to meeting this challenge.[33]

September: reduce the use of your car by walking more or using public transport. This will also go towards the August challenge of taking more responsibility for your health.

October: turn your home thermostat down a few degrees lower. Just a few degrees drop will save you over £100 a year and reduce the consumption of energy nationally.[34]

November: try to reduce food waste to close on nil. Currently we waste over a third of our food. That would feed most of the undernourished or starving throughout the world.[35]

December: switch your car to any that reduces your fuel consumption. Today there is no technological reason why we cannot produce cars that will give over 100 miles per gallon, rather than 0 to 60mph in fewer second, even this will make a significant reduction in CO2 emissions. This needs to be the most important criteria for car purchase, not its sporty performance. [36]

"I am helping heal the Earth!"

Chapter 15

The Cosmic Connection

"To see the world in a grain of sand and heaven in a wildflower, hold Infinity in the palm of your hand and eternity in an hour."

William Blake (1757-1827)

The sun is the sustainer of life and without it we would perish. It is no wonder that people throughout history have viewed the sun as a deity. Over time our understanding of the sun may have changed but it has been associated with every religion or culture from earliest times.

The sun is the ultimate light source for all life on earth either directly from the daylight, or indirectly from ancient sunlight, from fossil fuels that are effectively reservoirs of ancient sunlight. Read "The Last Hours of Ancient Sunlight" by Tom Hartmann. An exception might be light derived from nuclear power, but this is a replication of the process going on in the sun derived from the elements of an even earlier time in the earth's history.

It's interesting to note that light has been depicted as part of our makeup in many old paintings and icons that show halos of light over the heads of the human figures. Either this arose from some mass hallucination amongst artists or there has always been an awareness of such ephemeral light arising from certain people.

All our language is filled with this conscious awareness, we speak of a wise person as "enlightened", modern Christianity repeatedly refers to our being filled with "the light of god", and when we get excited, we "light up" and so on. There is some evidence that the main information transmission in our bodies may not be via the nervous system but by far faster light transmission through an optic fibre system that might also explain the above artist paintings and much more.

For thousands of years man has held the belief that we are all influenced by the entire cosmos, the planets, and stars. This was the foundation of astrology, which has, in recent times, been regarded as unscientific and unworthy of serious attention. But is it not reasonable to accept that if our everyday lives are clearly influenced by the sun and the moon, why should there be no influence from other cosmic bodies near and far? It is noteworthy that no lesser person than Karl Jung, the famous psychologist, expressed considerable interest in astrology and developed his theory of archetypes, that have been a part of astrology throughout history. In recent years these two fields of study have been brought together with psychological astrology by Liz Green.[47]

The work of Dr. Rudolph Steiner expanded the concept of planetary influence even further with specific relationships that have been recorded for thousands of years. The Sun has been associated with gold and our human heart, the Moon with silver and growth forces, Venus with copper and fluid forces in the body, Mars with iron in the blood and ego forces, Saturn with lead and hardening forces and intellectual growth, and so on. This work is discussed in detail in the work of Rudolph Hauschka, a student of Rudolf Steiner in his book The Nature of Substance.[37]

In physiology, we are learning more and more about the effect of light on our health, from its impact on the production of vitamin D to our skin, on the effect on waking and sleeping patterns, light pays a key role in governing the circadian rhythm, the internal clock that keeps the body synchronised with a 24-hour solar day. This circadian system is responsible for range of bodily functions and for regulating key hormones, including those that control our sleep rate cycle, melatonin, our feelings of hunger and our ability to feel full from the hormone greling. Blue light before bedtime and night may be bad news; but blue light in the morning and during the day can have a beneficial effect on our health. Red light however makes people feel more alert during the day and at night without impacting their sleep cycles. When residents at nursing homes and assisted living facilities, often exposed to constant dim light 24 hours a day, by simply giving them a robust light/dark pattern, dramatic improvements to their health and well-being are seen.

Modern man has, until recent health concerns about the dangers of overexposure to sun, enjoyed sunbathing as an essential ritual of summer holidays, often travelling abroad to ensure plenty of sunshine.

The use of light and particularly sunshine as a therapy has a long tradition, and in the early 1900s it was the mainstay for treatment of TB in many sanatoriums. In more recent times doctors have used the limited spectrum of natural light, ultraviolet, to treat many skin disorders and the use of light in winter months is used to treat SAD, associated with low levels of sun in northern hemispheres.

Quantum physics is changing our understanding of the universe and its impact on our lives, especially on the subject of consciousness. The idea that our brains are simply powerful computers that house all our thoughts, to the view that our brains are linked with a universal consciousness. The old Newtonian universe is being replaced with a far more mysterious, spooky one with the latest scientific research. Remember we are all made of stardust! The interstellar dust over aeons of time formed our solar system, our earth, and you and I! How did the random chaos of the Universe bring forth such miraculous order?

The Learning Universe and You

I started my further education studying physics at Birmingham University because I was very interested in nuclear physics, but after the first year I was asked to move on as I failed to pass the qualifying exams. My next choice of study was, it seemed at the time, as far from my first passion as could be imagined, psychology is what I wanted to read at university. Fortunately, or not, I could not get the support for this and finished studying a "useful subject", economics with statistics and accountancy at Hull University.

My career since then has taken many twists and turns but today I find myself in the health and medical profession and realise that those two young passions of physics and psychology were not so far apart as I once thought!

That question of "what was there before The Big Bang" (a question that even a five-year-old might ask) has always bothered me to a point that I had to find an answer, at least to satisfy myself, if no one else, especially as I have become convinced there is no separation between the universe and you and me.

1. My answer begins with a mind experiment. This was a favourite tool of Einstein when dealing with knotty problems such as the speed of light, when he visualised travelling on a beam of light himself!
2. Imagine an equilateral triangle, a very simple form, it may be a few centimetres across. Now expand it in your imagination first to as large as you wish, then reduce it to a point, all the time it is still an equilateral triangle. When it is just a point however it takes up no space, but it still bears the information of the triangle and exists in a timeless state, it can reappear at any time in any size. What has survived this "Alice in Wonderland Shrinking" is the information of an equilateral triangle.
3. Einstein gave us this wonderful simple formula for converting matter into energy and vice versa, $E=MC^2$ This means that the very small amount of matter can be converted into a vast amount of energy or vice versa, C being a very large number, 186,000 miles per second.
4. So, I thought I might use a similar conversion formula with a similar number but this time it would be about the conversion of information into energy and vice versa $I = ES^2$, where S is another very large number like C. This would mean a very small amount of energy could be converted into a vast amount of information and vice versa. It is not unreasonable to assume there would need to be some energy to hold that equilateral triangle information even when it was reduced to a point of no dimension.
5. Now comes the best part of the mind experiment. Now I ask you to convert all the matter in the universe, including yourself I'm afraid, into energy using Einstein's formula $E=MC^2$. You now have a universe composed only of energy.

Now would you convert all that energy into information using my hypothesised formula $I = ES^2$. You now have a universe devoid of stars, matter, energy, light and composed only of information.
6. Information needs no space or time to exist, could this be an alternative to The Big Bang. Could this be the" Zero Still Point"?
7. Immediately this information begins another cycle of condensation into energy, the energy into matter and the next universe as we know it comes into existence a universe filled with matter, energy, and information repeating unending cycles of expansion and contraction from form to information and back.

Where do you fit into this picture? All life involves increasing information or form. We speak of forming something. We are all being formed or informed from random chaotic particles. This is a process common to all living organisms, it is the reverse of entropy, the loss of form and pattern.

Many non-living things exhibit this forming process; when crystals are formed, when spiral galaxies are formed, when material atoms are formed. Where does the information come from for a rose or pine tree to grow? Is it really all in the genes or do the genes just carry the basic information of the building materials, the colour, scent, and cellular components. Is the design received from beyond, perhaps the gene is acting as an aerial receiving a "rose information" signal?

The shape of fir trees reminds one of the old-style TV aerials aimed at receiving fir tree signals from the informing universe! We live in an informing universe, and you and I are an integral part of that learning process.

The universe is constantly learning through every cycle of expansion and contraction. What we think, what we do, and the way we change the environment about us, all add to this process and leave a permanent mark on the universe forever. The religious might say the 'Zero Still Point' or pure information is the mind of God or Allah, others may see it as the conscious mind of the universe which we are all informing, and in turn are all formed by it as well.

"I Am the Universe, and the Universe is Me!"

Chapter 16

Facts & Figures

From "How Not to Die"

Michael Greger M.D.

As modern medicine is dominated by pathology I have focussed on health and the study of health in this book. It may be informative to look briefly at the major causes of our mortality, but at the same time recognise that usually it has been our lack of a healthy lifestyle that results in the increasing rarity of "death from old age" as opposed to death from some chronic disease. It is said that in some primitive societies the commonest cause of death is old age, but these societies are becoming few and far between as modern living takes its toll. The statistics below are from the most highly developed, most highly technologically organised, most medically advanced, and amongst the unhealthiest nations in the world, namely from the USA.

Mortality in the United States

		Annual deaths
1	Coronary heart disease	375,000
2	Lung diseases (lung cancer, COPD & Asthma)	296,000
3	You will be surprised!	225,000
4	Brain diseases (stroke and Alzheimer's)	214,000
5	Digestive cancers (colorectal, pancreatic & esophageal)	106,000
6	Infections (respiratory & blood)	95,000
7	Diabetes	76,000
8	High Blood Pressure	65,000
9	Liver disease (cirrhosis & cancer)	60,000

10	Blood cancers (Leukaemia, lymphoma & myeloma)	56,000
11	Kidney diseases	47,000
12	Breast cancer	41,000
13	Suicide	41,000
14	Prostate cancer	28,000
15	Parkinson's disease	25,000
	Total of all the above	1,750,000

What are the possible lifestyle factors that gave rise to these deaths?

1. Coronary heart disease- Main causes are diet and stress.
2. Lung diseases (lung cancer, COPD & asthma)- Main causes, smoking, diet, stress & poor breathing.
3. *You will be surprised!* - Main cause, iatrogenic or, in other words, medicine.
4. Brain diseases (stroke and Alzheimer's)- Main causes diet, stress, and lack of exercise.
5. Digestive cancers (colorectal, pancreatic & oesophageal)- Main causes diet, stress, and smoking
6. Infections (respiratory & blood)- Main causes diet, and stress
7. Diabetes- Main causes, diet, and stress.
8. High Blood Pressure- Main causes diet, stress, lack of exercise and salt
9. Liver disease (cirrhosis & cancer)- Main causes diet, stress, and alcohol
10. Blood cancers (Leukaemia, lymphoma & myeloma)- Main causes diet, and stress.
11. Kidney diseases- Main causes diet, and smoking
12. Breast cancer- Main causes diet, and lack of exercise.
13. Suicide- Main causes diet, mental stress, and lack of exercise.
14. Prostate cancer- Main causes diet, and lack of exercise.
15. Parkinson's disease- Main causes food, environmental toxins, and pollutants.

From the above table the two shocking conclusions are that almost 15% of all deaths are caused by medical treatment and that most of the rest, 85% of deaths are caused by or strongly associated with diet.

The outrage is made worse by the fact that most patients are not even told by their doctors that they can dramatically reduce most health risks with an improved diet, and that in many cases it is because their doctor didn't even know that, because it is not a significant part of their medical training. Yet another reason why we should all become, "Our own Doctor of Health and Happiness!"

Chapter 17

Swimming Against the Tide

"I don't mind dying, I just don't want it to be my fault!"

Dr. Kim Williams (Former President of the American College of Cardiology)

"Example is not the main thing influencing others; it's the only thing". Albert Schweitzer (1875-1965)

There is a powerful tidal wave that is man-made, that is an unexpected and undesirable product of our progress, economic policies, technology, and our mis-information age. We are all liable to be swept along with this all-pervading force unless we individually take on a greater responsibility to "swim against this tide".

It would be foolish to suggest all our progress over the past few hundred years has been harmful to the health of man and the planet, but a great deal has been. There may be many good reasons offered as to why this has happened; the pursuit of profit, greed with the desire to consume more rather than just enough, the excessive power of the media, our basic health education, and so on, but the main cause may have been something far simpler. The dominance of "Reductionism" over "Wholism" and Materialism over Consciousness.

I don't believe this tidal wave can be changed by governments alone but will require every one of us to cease "going with the flow, paddling happily and mindlessly with it", and by becoming more individually responsible for our own lives, our own health and the health and sustainability of our planet and all its flora and fauna. We all have, as a surviving species, the gift of response-ability, now we must all learn to use it. You and I can start to change our lifestyles and as this awakening of self-responsibility (remember the morphic resonance effect!) gathers momentum it will change the world for better and mankind will have a sustainable planet and a better future for our children and grandchildren.

"*I am a strong swimmer!*"

Afterword

You now have many ideas of ways to improve your health and wellbeing with lifestyle changes and the choice is yours.

Taking more care of your mechanics and body will impact on every aspect of your health. This was the basis of osteopathy when founded by Andrew Taylor Still and developed further by J M Littlejohn. When Littlejohn was asked," What are the limits of osteopathy?" His answer was brief and to the point - "No one knows". The limits are set by the patient and the practitioner.

As regards the significance of diet, the evidence is that most chronic diseases are closely linked if not entirely due to what we eat. The good news is that we can benefit from improved diet at any stage of our lives, *often even reversing established diseases.*

The rewards of improved breathing are almost as great as improved diet. The majority of the us breathe badly and suffer from some degree of chronic hidden hyperventilation and the many adverse effects due to this. As we improve our breathing there are two major benefits, improved tissue oxygenation and better control over the impact of modern stresses and anxiety. From my own research it also appears that breathing quality and diet quality are closely linked. As we improve one the other improves.[49]

Work on our mental outlook and our programmed sub-conscious mind can transform our lives. At its simplest level it means being positive about ourselves, never beating ourselves up, but learning to love ourselves for the miracle that we truly are.

Engaging with others in our community and recognising we are all one mankind whatever nationality, religion, ethnic group, or background we may have, will be the support we all need to deal with life's challenges. No man is an island, we are one family on this planet - "mankind".

Concern for our immediate environment and the larger environment of our planet will lead to a growing respect for this unique living entity called Gaia. We are a part of it and, the closer we get to realising this the healthier we shall be.

The biggest question often comes at the end of any discussion. "What are we?" Are we a part of a universal consciousness and not just an insignificant little machine that wears out and finishes up as dust? Modern science is beginning to favour the former concept. Do you?

Are you any wiser? Have you had any inspiring revelations? Are you more motivated to take up the challenge? Is your life's journey direction clearer? There seem to be two highways into the future, the further expansion and widening of the technological, reductionist, pathological highway of medicine as we know it today or the myriad of small lanes and minor roads that each traveller takes with self-responsibility for their own lives.

The former, as the saying goes is, "The road to Hell paved with good intentions", the latter could be the awakening of a new era of enlightenment and a kind of "Heaven on Earth!" The choice is ours!

"I am wiser and healthier every day!"

References:

1 Blue zones. Wikipedia, https://en.m.wikipedia.org/wiki/Blue_zone2

2 The World's Healthiest & Unhealthiest Countries, https://www.statista.com/chart/30313/health-and-healthcare-systems-index-scores/

3 What is Health? Harald Brussow, https://doi.org/10.1111/1751-7915.12063

4. The Evolving Role of Public Health in Medical Education, https://www.ncbi.nlm.nih.gov/pmc/articles/PMC7344251/

5. Connection-"Towards a broader understanding of health in Medicine", https://www.lulu.com/shop/michael-lingard/connection/paperback/product-23193878.html?page=1&pageSize=4

6.The Biology of Belief, Bruce H Lipton,
ISBN 0-97599147-7-7

7. Health education in medical training. At the time of writing, I have not been able to find any authorative statement on the proportion of a doctor's medical training devoted to health promotion & education. This alone tells us how low a priority "health" is in medical training. There are estimates of the time allocated to individual health education and promotion for patients representing just a few hours in a course lasting four years. Most attempts to improve this extraordinary imbalance tends to add "preventative medicine" to the course, more pathology orientated education of our doctors!

8. How Not to Die, Michael Greger M.D., Chapter 15.   Video talk: https://youtu.be/7rNY7xKyGCQ?si=ez-UXawwjnTcoGJ3

9. Connection, Towards a broader understanding of health in medicine.
https://www.lulu.com/shop/michael-lingard/connection/paperback/product-1p7dz79w.html?q=Connection&page=1&pageSize=4

10. An Overview of Osteopathic Medicine, Emil P. Lesho, DO
Arch Fam Med 1999;8:477-484

11. You Are the Placebo, Dr. Joe Dispenza, p84, Chap. 4

12. Quantum Body, Deepak Chopra,
ISBN 978-1-84604-769-5

13. The Science Delusion, Rupert Sheldrake.
ISBN 978-1-444-72792-0

14. Health and a Day, Lord Horder, Published by J M Dent in 1938, in Aldine Library series

15. The Body Connection, e-Book,
https://book.designrr.co/?id=20551&token=3168720268

16. You're Not Sick You're Thirsty, Dr.Batmanghelidj
ISBN 0-446-69074-0

17. The China Study, by Dr. T. Colin Campbell Ph.D,
ISBN 978-1932100-389

18. The Buteyko Guide to Better Breathing and Better Health, by Michael Lingard,
ISBN 978-0-244-77577-3

19. Spontaneous Evolution, Bruce.H.Lipton Ph.D: Chap.1. p8-26

20. Cured, Dr Jeff Rediger: ISBN 978-0-241-32755-5

21. Curing the Incurable, Dr Jerry Thompson:
ISBN 978-1-7816-176-0

22. Awareness Through Movement, The Feldenkraus Method.
ISBN 0-06-062344-6

23. Being Me and Also Us, Alison Stallibrass
ISBN 0-7073-0599-3

24. The Hidden Messages in Water, Dr. Masaru Imoto
ISBN 1-58270-114-8 p95

25. The Hidden Messages in Water, Dr. Masaru Imoto
ISBN 1-58270 pp.76-78

26. The Plastic Problem, https://4ocean.com

27. Local Produce, https://foodrevolution.org/blog/why-buy-local-food/

28. Overconsumption, https://www.ecowatch.com/overconsumption-fast-fashion-2399956999.html

29. Tree Planting, https://carbonfootprint.com/plantingtrees.html

30. Local Community, https://groundwork.org.uk

31. Why I Don't Eat Much Meat, Fish or Dairy,
https://www.youtube.com/watch?v=wRmo6VNjLCk&feature=youtu.be

32. Conserve Fresh Water, https://friendsoftheearth.uk/sustainable-living/13-best-ways-save-water

33. Make Your Health Your Responsibility,
https://totalhealthmatters.co.uk/

34. Thermostat, https://lifehacker.com/five-reasons-you-should-lower-your-thermostat-backed-b-1525010287

35. Food Wastage, https://olioex.com/food-waste/food-waste-facts/

36. Car Economy, https://www.whatcar.com/best/real-mpg-most-efficient-cars/n14356

37. The Nature of Substance, Rudoph Haushka,
ISBN 978-1-85584-122-2

38. You Are the Universe, Deepak Chopra
ISBN 978-1-84604-530-1

39. Knives over Forks! Video Trailer,
https://www.youtube.com/watch?v=O7ijukNzlUg

40. The Food Connection e-Book,
https://book.designrr.co/?id=27862&token=610166338

41. Morphic Resonance, Rupert Sheldrake
ISBN 978-159477317-4

42. Whole, by Dr. T Colin Campbell
ISBN 978-193785624-3

43. The Science Delusion, by Rupert Sheldrake
ISBN978-1-444-72792-0

44. https://thinkbynumbers.org/category/health/

45. Check Your Control Pause, Video timer:
https://youtu.be/JoKJ-FDbFlE?si=j8ip74odUcvAd3WD

46. PSYCH-K Centre International, https://psych-k.com/

47. Centre for Psychological Astrology https://www.cpalondon.com

48. Changing the programme in your sub-conscious.
https://youtu.be/GjcuD_Y9w9U?si=yVY7XsC8znGqrRBj

49. The Link between Diet & Breathing
https://totalhealthmatters.co.uk/the-relationship-of-diet-and-breathing/

50. The Pisa Pelvic Exercise, Podcast
Https://yourhealthinyourhands.simplecast.com/episodes/the-pisa-pelvic-exercise

51. The Food Connection eBook
https://book.designrr.co/?id=27862&token=610166338

52. The Role of Epigenetics in the Obesity Epidemic

https://youtu.be/3ckimoZ9BW4?si=OrmUNvEwteORX_4D

53. Recognising Health, Kenneth Barlow
ISBN 0-9513171-0-5

Reading List:

As I said at the start, we are all grateful reapers of the harvest planted by our fellow men and women who have often spent their lifetime trying to learn more for our benefit today and in the future. In early man this knowledge and wisdom was handed down by word of mouth but today we have the written word. Below I have listed some of the many books that have enriched my life, understanding, and knowledge.

4LeafGuide   Graff & Hicks   ISBN 978-1-5076-1341-2

A Model of Health   Roy Gillett   ISBN 0-947-878-25-4

A New Renaissance   David Loriman   ISBN 978-086315-759-2

Ageless Body Timeless Mind   Deepak Chopra   ISBN 0-7126-5673-1

Alexander Technique   Glynn MacDonald   ISBN 0-00-713385-5

Anthroposophical Medicine   Dr. Michael Evans   ISBN 0-7225-2771-3

Awareness Through Movement   Moshe Feldenkrais

ISBN 0-06-062344-6

Bees   Rudolf Steiner   ISBN 0-88010-457-0

Being Me and Also Us   Alison Stallibrass   ISBN 0-7073-0599-3

Beyond Matter Dr. Okiver Lazasr   ISBN 978-3039-330-270

Biology of Belief   Bruce Lipton   ISBN 0-9759914-7-7

Breaking the Food Seduction   Neal Barnard   ISBN 987-0312-31494-1

Catching The Light   Arthur Zajonc   ISBN   0-19-509575-8

Chaos   James Gleick   ISBN   978-0-718-18565-5

Climate change   Prince of Wales   ISBN   978-0-718-18565-5

Coming Home to Self   Nancy Verrier   ISBN   978-1-905664-81-8

Connection – Towards a broader understanding of... M Lingard

 ISBN   978-1-326-94022-5

Conversations with God   N D Walsch   ISBN   0-340-76544-5

Cracked   James Davies   ISBN   978-1845831556-3

Cured   Dr Jeff Rediger   ISBN 978-0-241-32755-5

Curing the Uncurable   Dr. Jerry Thompson ISBN 978-1-78161-176-0

Disease Proof   David L Katz   ISBN   978-1-59463-124-5

Disease Proof Your Child   Dr Joel Furman   ISBN   978-0-312-33808-4

Dr Neal Barnard's Reversing Diabetes   Dr Neal Barnard

ISBN   978-1-59486-810-8

Dr Neal Barnard's Cookbook Diabetes   Dr Neal Barnard

ISBN   978-1-62336-929-3

Emotional Intelligence   Daniel Goleman   ISBN 0-7475-2830-6

Eradicate Asthma Now - With Water   Dr. Betmanjeldi

ISBN   1-903571-354-9

Fit Baby, Smart Baby, Your Baby   Dr Glenn Doman

ISBN   978-0-7570-0376-9

Foodwise   Wendy E Cook   ISBN   978-1-905570-23-2

Forks over Knives   The Cookbook   Del Sroufe

ISBN   61519-187-1-061-4

Forks over Knives   Gene Stone   ISBN   978-1-6119-045-4

Frogs into Princes (NLP)   Richard Bandler   ISBN   0-911226-18-4

Full Planet, Empty Plates   Lester R Brown   ISBN   978-0-393-34415-8

Fundamentals of Therapy   Rudolph Steiner   ISBN   0-000-000-000

Fuzzy & Neuro Fuzzy Systems   Teodorescu   ISBN   0-8493-9806-1

Gaia   James Lovelock   ISBN   978-0-19-878488-3

Gut Bliss   Robynne Chutkan   ISBN   978-1-58333-551-2

Health and a Day   Lord Horder   ISBN   0-000-000-0

Healthy Eating Healthy World   J. Morris Hicks   ISBN   978-193666104-6

Holistic Cancer Medicine   Henning Saupe MD   ISBN 978-1-64502-155-1

How Not to Die   Dr Michael Greger   ISBN   978-1-250-06611-4

How Not to Die Cookbook   Dr Michael Greger

ISBN 788-1-50984-433-3

How the leopard …. (Peckham)   Brian Goodwin   ISBN   0-75380-171-x

How to give your baby….   Glen Doman   ISBN   0-7570-0376-9-182-6

How to Know Higher Worlds   Rudolph Steiner   ISBN   0-88010-372-1

How to Multiply Baby's Intelligence   Dr Glenn Doman

ISBN   978-1-910496-29

How to Teach Your Baby Math   Dr Glen Doman   ISBN   0-7570-0189-0

Hyperventilation Syndrome   Dinah Bradley   ISBN   1-85626-295-2

I Ching   Sam Reifler   ISBN   0-553-13677-

Life Lessons   E Kubler-Ross   ISBN   0-7432-0811-0

Love, Medicine and Miracles   Bernie Siegel   ISBN   0-7126-7046-7

Made for Goodness   Desmond Tutu   ISBN   978-006-170660-8

Medicine - Mythology & Spirituality   Dr R Twentyman

ISBN   1-85584-182-7

Milk The Deadly Poison   Robert Cohen   ISBN   0-9659196-0-9

Morphic Resonance   Rupert Sheldrake   ISBN   978-159477317-4

Natural Grace   Rupert Sheldrake   ISBN   0-385-48356-2

Nature Cure   Henry Lindlahr   ISBN   1-59224-070-4

Natures Alchemist   Anna Parkinson   ISBN   978-0-7112-2767-5

Plant Based Cookbook   T Sebben-Krupka   ISBN   978-0-2412-3003-9

Plant Powered Families   Dreena Burton   ISBN   978-1-941631-04-1

Quantum Shift in the Global Brain Ervin Laszlo ISBN 978-159477233-7

Quantum Body Deepak Chopra   ISBN978-1-84604-5

Recognising Health Kenneth Barlow ISBN 0-9513171-0-5

The Field of Form   Lawrence Edwards   ISBN0-903540-509-9

The Living Universe   Gary E Schwartz Ph.D ISBN 1-57174-455-x

The Low Carb Fraud   T Colin Campbell   ISBN   978-194035309-7

The Last Hours of Ancient Sunlight   Thom Hartmann

ISBN 978-0340822432

The Master & His Emissary   Ian McGilchrist   ISBN 978-0-300-24592-9

The Microbiome Diet   Raphael Kellman   ISBN   978-0-7382-1811-3

The Microbiome Solution   Robynne Cutkan   ISBN   978-1-58333-576-5

The Nature of Substance   Rudolf Hauschka   ISBN 978-1-85584-122-2

The New McDougall Cookbook   Dr John McDougall

ISBN   0-525-93610-6

The Patient Not the Cure   Dr M G Blackie   ISBN   0-356-08312-8

The Pleasure Trap   Douglas J Lisle   ISBN   978-1-57067-197-5

The Reverse Diabetes Diet   Dr Neal Barnard   ISBN   978-1-905744-57-2

The Salt Fix   Dr J Dinicolantonio   ISBN   978-0-349-41738-7

The Science Delusion   Rupert Sheldrake   ISBN 978-1-444-72792-0

Science Synthesis & Sanity   G. Scott Williamson & Innes Pearse

ISBN 0-7073-0259-5

Spontaneous Evolution   Bruce Lipton Ph D   ISBN 1-84850-305-2

The Starch Solution   Dr J McDougall   ISBN   978-1-60961-393-8

The Systems View of Life   F Capra & P Luisi   ISBN   978-1-107-01136-6

Vaccination   Viera Scheibener   ISBN   0-646-15124-x

Water Cures: Drugs Kill   F. Batmanghelidj MD   ISBN 0-9702458-1-5

Ways to go Beyond   Rupert Sheldrake   ISBN 978-1-473-65343-6

What is Wisdom   Cyril Upton   ISBN   978-0900001024

Whole   T Colin Campbell   ISBN   978-193785624-3

Why Zebras Don't Get Ulcers   Sapolsky   ISBN   0-7167-3210-6

Wine is the Best Medicine   Dr. Maury   ISBN   0-285-62250-1

You Are the Universe   Deepak Chopra   ISBN   978-1-84604-530-1

You Are the Placebo   Dr Joe Dispenza   ISBN 978-1-78180-257-1

You're Not Sick You're Thirsty!   Dr. Batmanghelidj

ISBN 0-446-69074-0

Your Body's Many Cries for Water   F Batmanghelidj

ISBN 0-9702458-8-2

Index

4LeafSurvey	37
Acupuncture	10
Albert Einstein	61
Albert Schweitzer	17
Alexander Technique	10
Alison Stallibrass	63
Allah	76
Alzheimer's Disease	37
Ancient sunlight	72
Andrew Taylor Still	83
Angina	51
Archetypes	73
Arterial circulation	32
Arthrtitis	37
Asthma	51
Astrology	72
B12	42
Bacteria	18
Being Me and Also Us	63
Big Bang	74
Birmingham university	74
Blood cancers	79
Blood pressure	37
Bloomberg Global Health Index	12
Body mechanics	30
Brain diseases	79
Breast cancer	79
Calcium	42
Calories	42

Cancer	23,37
Captain	23
Car emissions	71
Carbon dioxide	50
CHHV	51
Childhood development	63
Childhood memory	58
Cholesterol	42
Chronic hidden hyperventilation	51
Circadian rhythm	73
Colic	33
Community	70
Connection	16
Consciousness	47,57,81
Consumption of "Stuff"	69
Control Pause	51
Coronary heart disease	79
Cosmos	72
Counselling	58
Cowper	9
Crowded teeth	33
Dairy	33
Dehydration	44
Diabetes	37,43,79
Digestive cancers	79
Doctor	11
Doctor of Health & Happiness	11,24,60
Dr F Batmanhelidj	44
Dr F W Peabody	15
Dr Glenn Doman	63
Dr Innes-Pearce	62

Dr J Martin Littlejohn	20
Dr Kim Williams	81
Dr Rupert Sheldrake	47
Dr Scott-Williamson	66
Dr. T Colin Campbell	30
Drug therapy	31
Eating habits	39
Einstein	75
Electrocardiograph	23
Energy	75
Environment	66
Environmental damage	68
European School of Osteopathy	10
Evolution	26
Fake it till you make it	60
Fat	42
Fibre	42
Fight/Flight	60
Fizzy drinks	38
Food waste	70
Forks over Knives	41
Fresh water	70
Galaxies	76
Gastric reflux	51
General practitioner	23
Genes	17
God	76
Grains	38
Gravity	36
Greenhouse gases	70
Greling	73

Group practices	22
Guide to Water Needs	46
Habitat	68
Hale	63
Half a billion breaths	49
Hay fever	51
Healing	10
Health & a Day	20
Health of society	10
Health promotion	29
Health risk	39
Healthiest societies	11
Healthy Planet	69
Heaven on Earth	84
Herbal medicine	10
High blood pressure	79
Hippocrates	37
Holistic medicine	48
Homoeopathy	10,46
How not to die	78
Hull university	74
Hunter-gatherer	27
Hypnosis	58
Iatrogenic diseases	79
Immune system	48
Incurable diseases	28
Infections	79
Inflammation	23
Information	75
Information processing	57
Innate wisdom	67

Intelligence	73
J M Littlejohn	83
Karl Jung	73
Kidney disease	37,79
Lao Tzu	44
Leonardo da Vinci	63,67
Levity	36
Liver disease	79
Liz Green	73
Local produce	69
Lord Horder	13
Lung cancer	79
Machine	20
Mahatma Gandhi	56
Masaru Emoto	46
Mass	75
Materialism	81
Meat	38
Melatonin	73
Memories	58
Mental health	68
Mental tension	53
Michael Greger	78
Michelin Guide	9
Migraine	33
Milk replacements	41
Mind	56
Mind experiment	75
Miracle	26
Miraculous body	36
Miraculous machine	25

Morphic fields	47
Morphic resonance	82
Mortality	78
Muscle tension	53
New Year Resolution	69
Newtonian universe	73
NIH	14
Niko Tinbergen	61
NLP	58
Nocebo effect	56
Nursing homes	73
Nutrition	38
Nutrition therapy	10
Nuts & seeds	38
Oasis Reform	67
Optic fibres	72
Osteopath	10,20
Overconsumption	68
Paradigm shift	66
Parkinson's Disease	80
Pathology	29
Peckham Biologists	62
Pelvic torsion	33
Pharmaceutical industry	11
Physical therapy	32
Physics	74
Pisa Pelvic Exercise	34
Placebo effect	56
Plastic brain	56
Plastics	69
Pollution	68

Posture	35
Prof. Konstantin Buteyko	49
Prostate cancer	80
Protein	42
PSYCH-K	58
Psychology	74
Psychotherapy	4,53
Public transport	10,70
Quantum physics	18,74
Rainforests	69
Recipes	41
Reductionism	24,31,81
Replacement joint	33
Reprogramming the brain	59
Responsibility	15,26
Rob Williams	59
Royal Institute of Medicine	30
Rupert Sheldrake	67
SAD	74
Sea of oxygen	49
Shakespeare	9
Simple Guide to Healthier Eating	40
Snoring	51
Soul	18
Spain	12
Specialist	21
Spontaneous growth	65
Spontaneous remissions	28
Standard American Diet SAD	38
Steps	35
Stretching exercises	35

Stroke	37
Sub-conscious	57
Sub-occipital Release	34
Suicide	80
Symbiosis	18
TB	74
The China Study	38
The elephant in the healthcare room	49
The Hidden Messages in Water	46
The Peckham Experiment	61
The Sun	72
There is no such thing as Naughty	67
Thermostat	70
Tree planting	69
TV aerials	76
Universal consciousness	84
Variety of foods	41
Vegetables	38
Vegetarian diet	29
Vitamin D	42,73
Walking	35
Water	44
Wealden Clinic	10,21
What is Health?	13
Whole plant diet	38
Wholism	81
William Blake	72
Wisdom	9
Zero still point	76

Printed and bound by CPI Group (UK) Ltd, Croydon, CR0 4YY
06/08/2024
01024187-0004